Keeping Secrets and Telling Lies

Revealing the truth about disease
and Self-Healing!

Dr. Robert R. DeSantis

David Lloyd, B.M.E., CECP

MEDICAL DISCLAIMER

The information provided is for informational purposes only. The information in this book should not be a substitute for the advice of a qualified and licensed physician or other healthcare provider. In the event you use the information in this book for yourself, the authors and the publisher assume no responsibility for your actions.

The high priests refused to look through Galileo's telescope lens, for they were beyond scared to see the proof they were wrong.

Contents

Introduction

Over the last 150 years, we have skyrocketing amounts of cancer and disease that have never been known to man. Some say we have increased disease because we never had the proper testing. But the number of chronic illnesses and diseases that never existed 150 years ago, like autism, childhood cancer, diabetes and Alzheimer's, are not explained. Even 50 years ago, when we were kids, we didn't see classmates with autism or allergies or grandparents with diabetes or Alzheimer's. Cancer and infertility weren't common in every family. What has happened in the last 150 years that created such a decline in the health of the world and especially the United States?

The secrets we will share with you are so crucial to the health of you and your family that it's time they are revealed.

Health practices have deviated from what they used to be. The common practices for health back in the 1860s, which relied on hygiene, sanitation, diet and spirituality, were soon overshadowed by a diagnosis, a pill, a vaccination, and:

NOT A SPOILER ALERT – BIG PROFITS through Monopolies!

When Louis Pasteur propagated experiments with questionable data, soon a mercury pill and a vaccine were part of every medical doctor's prescription for public health!

Due to the startup of the American Medical Association (AMA) in 1847 and the propaganda they spread using smear campaigns, the doctors of the late 1800s and early 1900s that believed in natural cures of herbs, good hygiene, better nutrition, and energy healing became known as little more than witch doctors, quacks, and snake oil salesmen.

Big Pharma was ready to take over the profitable health industry, and anyone that opposed them was met with jail time or a shortened life span. Big Pharma even set up a committee within the American Medical Association (AMA) to discredit and eliminate anyone that caused potential competition to the almighty drug and vaccine monopoly. OK, did you raise your eyebrow? We encourage you to keep reading!

The Big Pharma monopoly and deceit are still going strong today. Big Pharma has pulled the wool over our eyes and *tricked* us into the fear of infectious diseases and cancer. If you raised your eyebrow, we will introduce you to Dr. Ignaz Semmelweis shortly.

The incredible disinformation and censorship, along with the actual permanent removal of individuals who have publicized success with diseases like cancer, is nothing less than crimes against humanity.

We are here to change that. We are on a mission. We are shifting the world into a whole new paradigm and expressing a new consciousness.

It's time you know their secrets!

"An error does not become truth by reason of multiplied propagation, nor does truth become error because nobody sees it" -Mahatma Gandhi

---

So, sit down, grab your favorite blanket, pull up a chair and get comfortable. Get ready to learn well-kept secrets, the tragedy of Dr. Semmelweis, crazy Aaron the Rock Star, and Aaron's genius backup singers. These secrets will affect what you do and think EVERY SINGLE DAY. We all know it's no secret that Big Pharma makes a lot of money by charging large sums and NOT "finding cures" as they are forever collecting money for their research. But you don't realize that they have been keeping some REALLY, REALLY BIG SECRETS!!

At the risk of sounding like complete wackos, we're hoping we can save more than a few lives!

So, did you pull up a chair yet? Well, hold onto your hat! Here we go...

Chapter 1
Do Germs Make Us Sick?

We have been repeatedly told that germs make us sick. We know it will take a lot of convincing for us to explain what germs are here for. Yes, they are everywhere. And, yes, germs can cause symptoms that make you feel sick. However, before we deep-dive into any of it, let's set the stage with a little story.

Imagine, if you would, you have a good friend that became a Rock Star. Let's call him Aaron. He traveled the world with his band, recording songs and singing at sold-out concerts. He has a multitude of fans, signed thousands of autographs, and makes millions of dollars every year. Aaron loves to wear outrageous and stylish clothing. It seemed as if the whole world was following him! People would dole out their money for anything he offered. And then, as he aged, he was on his deathbed. You visit him in the hospital, and you see him lying destitute on his hospital bed. He has a hospital gown on, and you notice his trademark gold necklace with the gold microphone pendant. Then Aaron reveals something that astounds you. He can barely talk, but he extends his hand to you and slowly places his golden necklace in your palm. He wearily looks out the window and sheepishly says, "I have a confession...it's hard to admit, but...I want you to know something..."

You ask him, "What? What are you trying to say?"

He slowly tells you, "Well...I have to be honest with you...I never really sang any of my songs, I was only lip-syncing. I crave attention and adore it when people follow me and spend money at my concerts."

And you ask him in astonishment, "Who sang the songs?"

He turns to you and answers, "It was Pierre, the lead backup singer. I only knew how to lip-sync."

How would you take that? What would you feel?

Back in 1895, something similar to that actually happened in the science community, and to this day, billions of lives have been adversely affected by it. There obviously weren't any Rock Stars back then, but there was a well-known scientist, Louis Pasteur, who had the same mindset throughout his career. He also made an astonishing confession about his life's work on his deathbed. Read the following quote:

"The germ is nothing, the terrain is everything." - Louis Pasteur (deathbed confession)

The first secret is that germs, bacteria, and fungi are not the bad guys. They *don't* make you sick. They support you in your health! We'll repeat, germs don't make us sick! The word "terrain" is originally a French word referring to everything: land, soil, surfaces, skin, table tops, floors, part of the whole, etc.

You might have shaken your head, maybe even rolled your eyes? It's OK. We will explain why coming up. Reading "germs don't make us sick" right at the beginning of this book may be hard to take in, but hang in there with us and keep reading! Dr. Semmelweis is on his way.

Why does this matter to you? To your kids? Your family? Because our entire medical industry is built on the hoax that germs (including viruses) make you sick! Germs have an *intrinsic purpose* in nature and biology and DO NOT make us sick. Understanding the truth that *germs don't make us sick* gives you one less thing to worry about. Now imagine all the people who, at this instant, after they read those last few sentences, let out a big sigh of relief and let go of their FEAR! We have so many drugs and vaccinations based on the Germ Theory, and they simply aren't necessary. Many drugs and vaccines are *harmful despite what we are told by slick TV commercials and Big Pharma-backed advertisement campaigns.* The list of ingredients that go into vaccines would make a Poison Control Center doctor go into a tizzy. The whole concept of the coronavirus is based on this hoax. (Eye roll?)

One of the first questions people are quick to ask is, "So, what is making us sick?" We will slowly reveal that answer after we give you the background on why we have been so *ingrained* to believe that germs make us sick. We will also explain why so many people died from the Coronavirus scare. Honest doctors, scientists, and psychologists are now understanding more clearly, what is happening in our bodies. They have found that a symbiotic relationship exists between germs and our terrain.

You may think this sounds crazy, which makes us sound crazy, but we're motivated to keep speaking the truth anyway. You may have popped your head back, rolled your eyes, and shaken your head in disbelief several times by now. If you did, it's the Semmelweis Reflex. We'll explain what that is in Chapter 3.

Hear us out! There is proof, and it all leads us back to Louis Pasteur.

There is now proof that Louis Pasteur INVENTED the Germ Theory using fudged numbers, fraudulent experiments, and fictitious findings! [1] Yes, there is *actual proof* that his private notes and experiments were fraudulent. We will explain more about this starting in Chapter 4.

Let's first look at what the Germ Theory is.

Chapter 2
What is the Germ Theory all about anyway?

The Germ Theory states that *diseases are caused by an invasion of germs*. But the **GERM THEORY IS NOT TRUE!** Louis Pasteur, known as the Father of the Germ Theory, was paid by the French government to go against the scientists of the day. How do we know this is true? Because his private experiment notes were finally released by his grandson in 1964 after being hidden since Louis Pasteur had written them. A book was published in 1995 called The Private Science of Louis Pasteur, by Gerald Geisen.[1] The book reveals all of Pasteur's notes and prove he falsified his experiment results. Most of his experiments were failures! Yet, he lied to the European people.

Before we get to all that, let us tell you a little bit about Louis…

The Amazing Story of "TRICKY" LOUIS PASTEUR

Now listen close…here's another little story. There once was a man named Louis Pasteur. Imagine Louis grew up wanting to be rich and famous. He wanted to be the Rock Star of his day! Sadly, he was not interested in truth, nor did he have much of a conscience. When Louis grew up, he decided to be a chemist. To make a long story short, starting in the 1860s, he was given A LOT of money and fame by the French government and church to go against the common scientific beliefs. The church had a tremendous influence on governments back in the late 1800s.

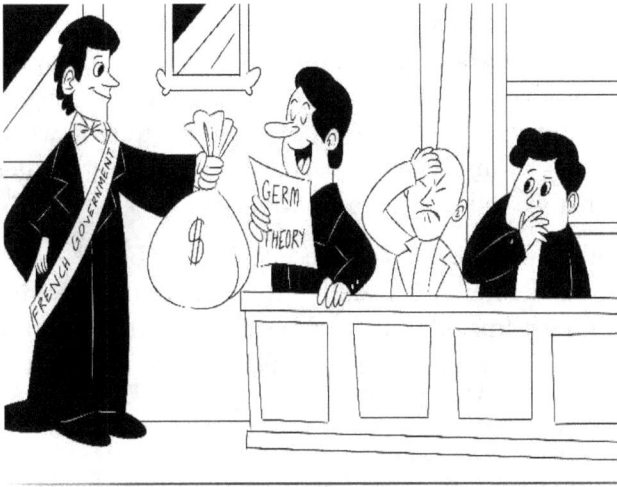

Stay with us here! Both the church and government wanted Louis Pasteur to "do research" in 1857 and prove that germs were not spontaneously created but that they came from the environment. This was called the *Germ Theory*. Some people took the hook, the line, and the sinker. It's become mass hypnosis. We are here to *question* it because so many people HAVEN'T!

"The bigger the lie, the more people will believe it." Joseph Goebbels

---

When our terrain (body) is altered by toxins such as chemicals or stress, *that's when* germs are utilized to get the body back into harmony. Essentially all DISEASE can be traced back to a DIS-EASE or a lack of ease. Or rather, some STRESS toxin that comes in a physical, mental, or spiritual form. We have all eaten chemicals, parasites, or drugs that change our terrain. Most of us have dealt with the stress of overeating. But what about a stress that resulted from a fight or a constant worry about a loved one? What about the stress that creates cancerous thoughts of anger, hatred, and resentment? What do these kinds of stresses do to our terrain (body)? How do you think our bodies react and repair the changes? This is where germs come into the picture. Germs are *utilized in the healing process* of the body terrain, which has been altered by stress toxins. This is the reason WHY we see germs in the vicinity of what we call disease in our bodies.

The assumption that germs are the enemy was based on the level of understanding our forefathers had. Unfortunately, that assumption is still perpetuated today! Imagine the world back in the 1800s, no internet, no air travel, no bullet trains, and no cell phones. The first phone was invented in 1876 by Alexander Graham Bell, and they were not widely used until the 1920s.

Go back in time even further. Think of how long it took humans to understand that the Earth IS NOT FLAT! It never has been. It took until the 17th Century for most people in the Asian part of the world to change their thinking about it! [2] Millions of people in early Asia undoubtedly shook their heads and rolled their eyes whenever someone brought up the idea that the Earth is round. The head jerk! Some people still believe the Earth is flat!

We ask that you have an open mind *and* heart, and let's all emerge from our collective ignorance-is-bliss syndrome.

- *"Ignorance is Bliss."* - Thomas Gray

Chapter 3
Who is Dr. Semmelweis, you ask?

Before we continue, you need to know about the Semmelweis Reflex. Some people have a tendency to say, "you're crazy and full of it!" when they hear something new that sounds contrary to what is accepted. We have seen people jerk their heads back in disbelief! This is where it is helpful to understand the Semmelweis Reflex.

Let us tell you the story of Dr. Ignaz Semmelweis. Dr. Ignaz Semmelweis was a Hungarian physician who discovered the importance of *hygiene* in 1847. He found that if doctors cleaned their hands after they did an autopsy and before they saw patients, many lives would be saved. Go figure! Now we practice it for many of our everyday situations, simply following our common sense. Dr. Semmelweis's studies on simply cleaning your hands before delivering a baby showed that that alone could reduce the death rate from 13% to less than 2%.

You would think he would be celebrated for his findings. But no! The opposite occurred. When Dr. Semmelweis presented his "revolutionary" findings to his colleagues hoping they would be implemented with enthusiasm, he found himself locked up for his "dangerous" ideas about hygiene!

Dr. Semmelweis was called *crazy* by his medical colleagues *and* *imprisoned* in an insane asylum for suggesting they all wash their hands before seeing patients! Sadly, he died just two weeks later. Can you imagine the shock he went through? Or the unexpected, isolating, and intense conflict he felt?

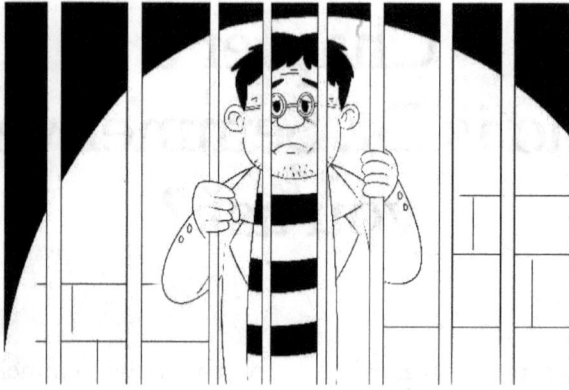

Get it? New ideas are not received well in the medical industry. By the public or media.

This is now called the **Semmelweis Reflex. There is a tendency to reject new evidence or new knowledge because it contradicts established norms, beliefs, or paradigms**. It took over 100 years for doctors to finally accept Semmelweis's findings!

We relate this because *you* may need to overcome your own Semmelweis Reflex.

You might say, "Well, of course, Semmelweis was washing off germs". However, germs are all over. They are part of the whole as Louis Pasteur finally confessed that he was wrong about claiming germs cause disease. Now that we know Pasteur's private science notes are nothing close to what was told to the public, we can view germs for their intrinsic purpose. The cells in our bodies *naturally make* germs for a reason! Germs can never be washed away. Germs are some of the smallest particles in our bodies.

Semmelweis was washing away bigger particles like dirt, grease, fecal matter, urine, toxins, and bodily fluids like blood! Those are the particles that make the body *react*. The body responds as if they are foreign intruders. Germs are not foreign intruders! Our cells actually *MAKE* germs and bacteria for a *purpose, which we will learn.*

Let's make a clarification between hygiene and sterilization. Hygiene is the cleansing of our environment. Sterilization is the killing of germs, bacteria, and fungi that are simply part of nature and harmlessly coexist with the whole. If someone must go into surgery after an accident, hygiene is always practiced. Sterilizing all the instruments is an *additional* step to have peace of mind from the perspective of the Germ Theory mentality we've all come to believe. Yes, we are happy that doctors and nurses are hygienically cleansing their workplaces. However, harmless germs, bacteria, and fungi are already part of the whole. They are not the bad guys! Resist your Semmelweis Reflex!

It is high time we embrace valid, proven science that has no open holes. We have a system that has answers that change depending on who is holding out the money. Our medical and science industries have been truly hijacked by unscrupulous professionals and CEOs, and we are paying ransoms every day with our health and our lives. Let's rewind our mentality and start anew.

Next, we'll look at the Spontaneous Generation Theory .

Chapter 4
What is Spontaneous Generation Theory?

"If I could live my life over again, I would devote it to proving that germs seek their natural habitat, diseased tissue – rather than being the cause of the diseased tissue."
- Rudolph Virchow

Virchow is known as "the father of modern pathology" and to his colleagues, the "Pope of medicine.".[3] Now picture Antione Bechamp (Pierre Jacques Antione Bechamp, 1816-1908), a humble and brilliant scientist and professor (1855). He was known for many *reproducible* experiments proving germs did not come from the air. He showed germs came from what he called Microzymas inside the organism. He called this new discovery *Spontaneous Generation* in 1855. *"Reproducible"* is the most important word in science. If experiments cannot be reproduced by other scientists, then theories are *proven false*!

Bechamp's experiments proved that an organism would produce a germ spontaneously if it were in the presence of something toxic or if dead cells needed to be decomposed. Other scientists like Claude Bernard and Guenther Enderlein were also validating these findings. Let's call them the backup singers of the late 1800s who were overshadowed by a flamboyant lip-syncing lead singer. If you're not familiar with anyone in the music industry, backup singers are highly respected because band mates know how much they add to the overall sound of a band.

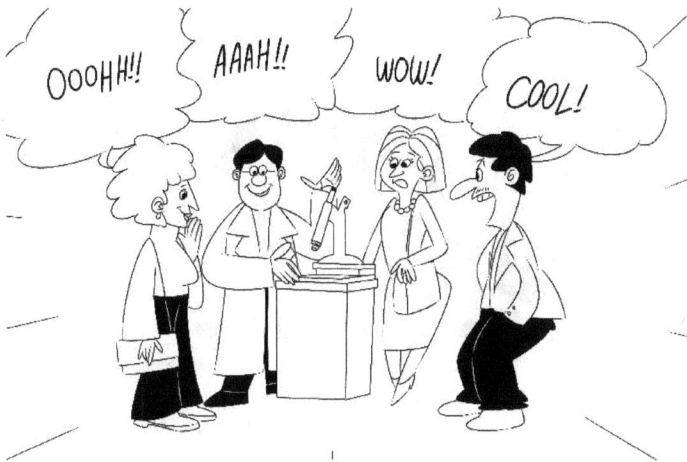

Strangely, the leaders of the French government and church didn't want the public to adopt the ideas of Bechamp and other famous scientists. *Spontaneous generation* means the body heals and protects itself. Yes, the body can heal and protect itself.

Did you shake your head again? Perhaps a Semmelweis Reflex?

The *Germ Theory* promotes the man-made idea that life itself is a *WAR* and we are always under attack from airborne germs. Spontaneous Generation Theory proved that *nature lives in harmony*. We are producing our own germs in order to support our health. *Nature always strives to create harmonious balance!*

To continue, "tricky" Louis (as he was nicknamed) was paid to make sure that scientists like Bechamp and their experiments were discredited. He was a great speaker and a convincing salesman. He spoke about his *personal* version of scien*ce full of fraudulent results*. And, helped by propaganda and government funding, he promoted his ideas far and wide (even though they were untrue).

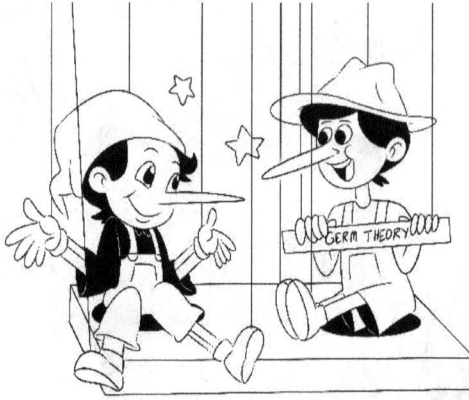

And what was he saying? Well, for starters, Louis Pasteur said that germs were causing disease and making people sick. And that you could use vaccinations to protect people from these diseases. Do you sense any ulterior motives that would have been at play?

Chapter 5
HOW DID THOSE PEOPLE GET BLOODY DIARRHEA?

Hey! We know that came out of left field, but just seeing if you are still with us! Louis Pasteur started off by saying that people were getting bloody diarrhea from a bacteria called listeria. He claimed that some cow's milk had been contaminated because the cows had the listeria bacteria, and now everyone that drank the milk was getting sick.

But get this! Listeria bacteria is found in HEALTHY cows. Also, listeria can be injected into healthy cows without causing any sickness to the cow or anyone else!

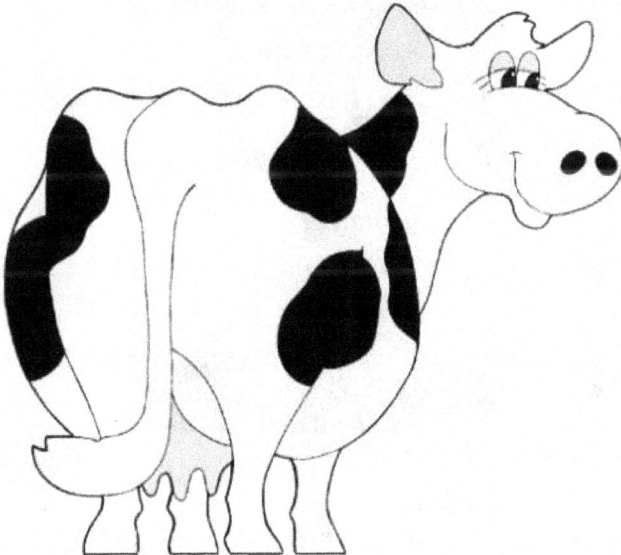

The truth of the matter is that listeria is *always* in a cow.

When the cow was taking in toxins from drinking water and food that was contaminated, then the cow's own milk was contaminated. To be specific, *listeria bacteria was <u>breaking down</u> the cells harmed by the toxins in the cow's body, and it came out in the milk.* The toxic milk was causing the problem.

Experimentally, listeria was not the cause of the bloody diarrhea. But that fact was hidden by Louis Pasteur's fraud. And thus began the war on bacteria, or at the very least, the **Germ Theory** was begun!

Here's an interesting excerpt from Dr. Tom Cowan, MD and Sally Fallon Morell's great book, The Truth About Contagion (originally titled The Contagion Myth). [4]

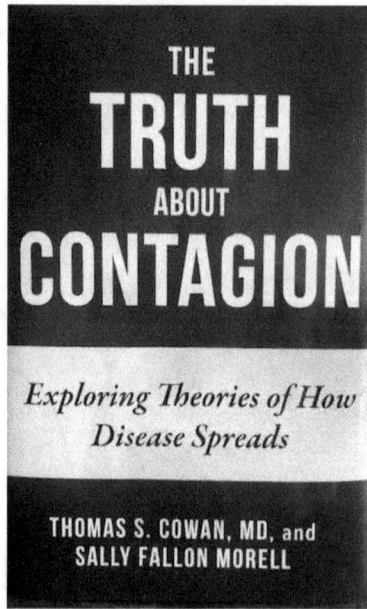

"Pasteur did this type of experiment for forty years. He found sick people, claimed to have isolated a bacterium, gave the "pure culture" to animals—often by *injecting it into their brains*—and made them sick. He became the celebrity scientist of his time, feted by kings and prime ministers, and hailed as a great scientist. His work led to pasteurization, a technique responsible for destroying the integrity and health-giving properties of milk. His experiments ushered in germ theory of disease..." [5]

"Since Pasteur's day, *no one* has demonstrated experimentally the transmissibility of disease with pure cultures of bacteria or viruses." [6]

Read on to find out why no one else could reproduce these experiments!

On his deathbed, Louis admitted that the whole effort to prove contagion <u>was a failure</u>, leading to his famous deathbed confession: **"The germ is nothing; the terrain is everything."** That concludes and proves *he MADE UP the findings that germs cause disease!! He made it up!! We all need to question it now.*

Unfortunately, Louis Pasteur's fraud never made it to mainstream news. To this very day, we have the belief that germs make us sick. We'll say it again: germs are not the bad guys!

Had anybody in power or with a voice in the media bothered to make sure that Louis had notes or experiments that backed up what he was saying, we would not have the incredible health problems of today. Unfortunately, *Tricky Louis, as he was called, would not let any of his notes or experimental results be seen by any of his coworkers, colleagues, or family members.* **He was very quick to discredit everyone else's work publicly, but he would not let anyone look at his own! His ego let him blatantly lie to the world.**

His whole life, Louis Pasteur would not let ANYONE read any of his notes or experiments ever! He made his family promise they would not release his notes even upon his death. Did you get that? He made his family promise not to release his private science notes even after he died!

It was well known that Louis *even* took his notes with him on vacation!! If they had airplanes back then, he would have been the guy sitting in first class with the black briefcase handcuffed to his left wrist.

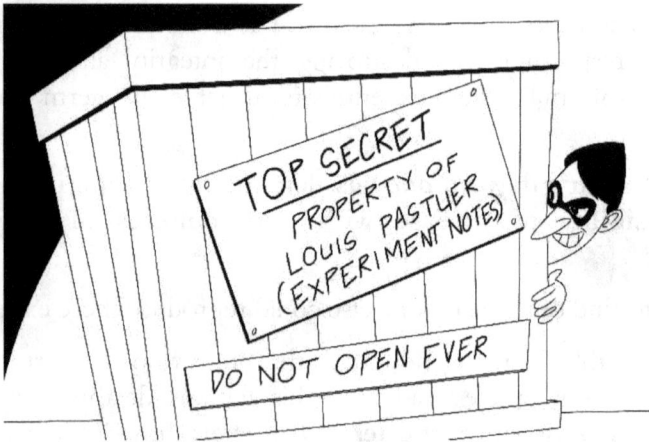

How do we know Louis Pasteur was making things up about his findings? Because Louis Pasteur's grandson, who was named in Louis' honor, Louis Pasteur Vallery-Radot, must have had a real conscience. He finally released his grandfather's notes in 1964. The notes were published in 1995. Gerald Geisen researched the published private notes of Louis Pasteur and wrote a book about the notes. In his book, *The Private Science of Louis Pasteur,* by Gerald Geisen, Geisen confirmed what was known by scientists like Bechamp all along...*that Louis Pasteur was a fraud and a phony!*

"There is no war going on between our cells in our body", Dr. Stephan Lanka, Renowned Virologist and Scientist, Freedom Talk 5.

In the notebooks, Pasteur states he could not transfer disease with a pure culture of bacteria. He would sometimes grind up the brains of animals and *inject* the mix into *the brain* of another animal to "prove" contagion. Or he would *add poisons* to his culture and then inject it to cause symptoms. Truly mad science!

Geisen writes, "The conclusion is unavoidable: *Pasteur deliberately deceived the public,*

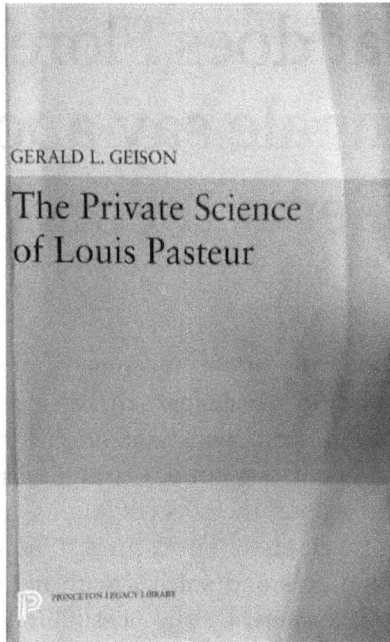

GERALD L. GEISON

The Private Science
of Louis Pasteur

PRINCETON LEGACY LIBRARY

including especially those scientists most familiar with his published work." The Private Science of Louis Pasteur by Geisen.[7] So, 150 years of fraudulent science has been promoted to the public for the sake of keeping people in the dark about their own power within! To this very day, Louis Pasteur is celebrated and written about as if he were a hero. And yet, *NOT ONE* of his experiments on Germ Theory or vaccines is *reproducible*. We will go into more detail about what was in his private notes in Chapter 8.

Chapter 6
What does Florence Nightingale say about the Germ theory?

Florence Nightingale, the most famous nurse in history, said, "There are no specific diseases: there are specific disease *conditions*." She says, "Is it not living in continual mistake to look upon disease as we do now, as separate entities, which must exist, like cats and dogs, instead of looking upon them as conditions, like a dirty and clean condition, and just as much under our control." She says of smallpox, "I have seen with my own eyes and smelled with my own nose smallpox growing up in where it *could not* by any possibility have been *caught* but must have *begun*." [8]

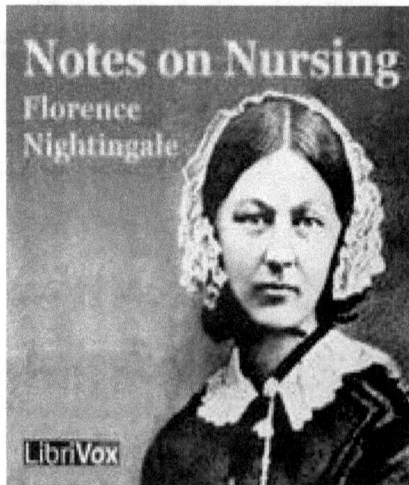

It's time to repeat these secrets the medical industry keeps well hidden. So well hidden that they still teach the Germ Theory in all schools!!

There is an overwhelming abundance of proof that the Germ Theory is a fraud and has been misleading us for 150 years. You only must be aware of the facts. Facts hidden in plain sight!

A good book to help you in your research is What Really Makes You Ill? Why Everything You Thought You Knew About Disease is Wrong by Dawn Lester and David Parker. [9] It has thousands of additional references beyond what we've listed in the back of this book, and it took ten years to write!

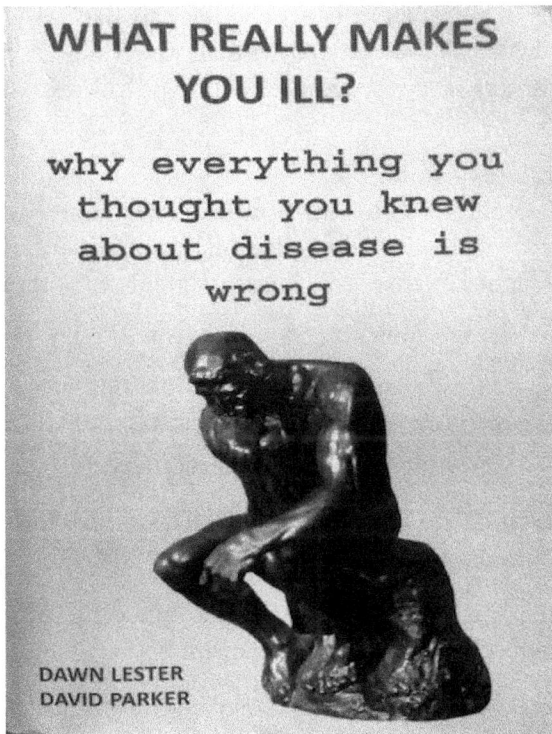

WHAT REALLY MAKES YOU ILL?

why everything you thought you knew about disease is wrong

DAWN LESTER
DAVID PARKER

Chapter 7
Disease Postulates and Raisin Wrinkles

Why is it that *not one* disease meets the criteria for infectious disease?

Where there is a Joker, there is a Penguin, ask Batman! Louis Pasteur was the Joker back in his day, along with another dubious character who came up with several *seemingly logical*, scientific postulates.

These notable offerings from science in the late 1800s are the famous **"Koch's postulates."** Robert Koch (who was also said to be crooked, or "Koched" lol) came up with four postulates which are very commonly known by most scientists and doctors as the *"gold standard"* for diagnosing infectious disease. We all learned them in biology class.

Here they are, there are four:

1. The germ must be found in abundance in <u>all</u> cases suffering from the disease but <u>NOT</u> found in <u>healthy</u> organisms. [Do you see why the COVID-19 testing seems a bit questionable?]

2. The ***germ must be isolated*** from a diseased organism and grown in a pure culture.

3. The isolated and cultured germ **should cause the original disease** when introduced into a healthy organism.

4. The isolated germs must be re-isolated from the now diseased organism which received the shot of isolated, cultured germs and identified as IDENTICAL to the original type of germ which was in the shot. [10]

And they make PERFECT sense. This is truly the only way to prove the causation of a germ. The crazy thing is that *not one disease* meets all four criteria!!

We'll say it again...Koch's Postulates are considered the "*gold standard*" for diagnosing a disease, and yet there is *no bacterial OR viral disease ever proven to meet the standards! However, there are a lot of fraudulent scientists claiming that they have...*

Let's look at our cells in a new light. Our cells know how to function without our interference. We have been taught there needs to be some "extra" assistance for our cells to stay healthy. We have been taught that our cells are under attack. Picture a human cell as a bowl of trail mix. Cells are full of all kinds of small parts. Think of those small parts as the peanuts, dried fruit, chocolate chips, and raisins in all kinds of tasty flavors and colors in the trail mix. There is nothing wrong with the glass bowl full of trail mix sitting on your kitchen table. We all love to snack!

Our now infamous "Aaron the Rock Star" loved trail mix. He had bowls of trail mix in his house, his studio, his car, everywhere. His own son had the same fondness for eating trail mix, too. (What kid wouldn't!) One day Aaron saw a big clump of raisins in the glass bottom of one of his trail mix bowls. He was puzzled how the raisins got stuck together. Odd. More oddly, he noticed raw brown sugar crystals in the wrinkled grooves of the raisins. After a few weeks of seeing those odd raisins in the bottom of the bowl, he convinced himself that the raisins should not clump together in trail mix.

Several weeks later, Aaron's son, Tiger, was on the sofa sulking. Aaron noticed his son's face was slightly red. Aaron asked, "Tiger, what's up with you?"

His son responded, "Don't call me Tiger anymore! I don't like that nickname anymore. In fact, I hate it now!"

Aaron asked, "What's wrong, you sound angry!"

Tiger said, "I am! That mean kid at school stole my football and kept telling his friends that he *just happened* to find it on the field two days ago.

It was my favorite football with the cool colors! Everyone else knows it's mine, but he won't give it back!!"

Aaron said, "We will talk to him and his parents to get to the bottom of it. We'll get your football back!"

His son said, "I doubt it! He is the biggest jerk in the school! I'm going downstairs to your music studio and pound on the drum set for a while! I don't want you to stop me!"

Aaron sighed and said, "Alright, but shut the door, please!"

After Tiger left, Aaron looked down on the table and saw four raisins left in that bowl of trail mix. He thought nothing of it at first. Maybe Tiger ate the clump of raisins along with some of the trail mix. Then, the next day, Tiger complained he was feeling sick to his stomach. Aaron thought his son *must* have eaten some clumped-up raisins! The raisins shouldn't be clumping in the trail mix. Something is wrong with raisins in trail mix. Aaron believed in his brain those raw brown sugar crystals were the suspicious culprits. He *knew* something wasn't right with raisins. Why are sugar crystals on the raisins? He started experiments to prove there must be something wrong with raw sugar crystals, especially the ones you see in the wrinkles of raisins. His curiosity started spinning!

He came up with the crazy idea that he could separate the smallest sugar crystals from the raisins and get more crystals to grow. He picked out three raisins with a sterilized spoon and placed them in another small clean bowl. He was certain that he would find more raw sugar crystals within a few days if he added more dried raisins and let them sit overnight. He planned to feed the new crystals to his dog to see if his dog would get sick.

No matter how hard he tried, he couldn't separate the crystals from the raisins. With everything he did, there always remained a small bit of raisin along with each crystal. And if the raisin bit was too small, the crystals would disappear. However, he was so convinced he could prove the raw sugar crystals were making people and animals sick, he told his bandmates, the backup singers, and his producer that raisins with raw sugar crystals in the wrinkles will make you feel queasy if you eat them.

Aaron was so charismatic that everyone believed he was onto something which would change the way people view raw sugar crystals. Aaron talked to his producer repeatedly and easily convinced his producer to give him weekly bonuses to further his experiments. Aaron kept his experiments going and took hundreds of notes, but he let no one see his notes! At every new city where he played a concert, he would talk with people in high positions. He tells everyone he has transferred bad sugar crystals from raisins in his lab experiments into other bowls of raisins and trail mix, and more bad sugar crystals appeared. In his loud-speaking voice, he proclaims to everyone he hasn't had any failures. He says he then fed the new sugar crystals to his dog, and his dog acted differently. Aaron claims he has successfully extracted raw sugar from raisins, and that is *precisely* what makes people and animals get sick. He tells people the results prove, without a doubt, that raw brown sugar crystals are DANGEROUS!

Aaron was constantly trying to prove his point. After talking about it for so long, he heard other people agree with him that raw brown sugar crystals are attacking the cells inside of our stomachs! Without even questioning his work! After all, he must be a genius because he is... a rock star. Before too long, everyone was describing raw sugar crystals as "DANGEROUS and DEADLY".

One night after a concert, his lead backup singer, Pierre, said he had been eating trail mix and raisins for a week, and he felt amazing. "They don't make me sick at all!" But Aaron quickly got on stage the next day and told the audience he was auditioning a new backup singer because his former backup singer had been lying to the band and wasn't prepared for rehearsals.

Later that night, Aaron was in his dressing room. He swiped everything off of his dressing table and hammered his fists on the top. He realized he could not fire Pierre! Aaron's mind was eating away at itself because he knew Pierre was the actual voice of the band. Pierre was the real reason everyone adored the band and made them famous.

Aaron would not admit that he could *NEVER* isolate the raw brown sugar crystals! His ego wouldn't let go of the secret. He was being paid amazing amounts of money. It's the kind of secret that if one talks about it enough, even though one knows it is incorrect, your ego would keep it secret until your deathbed...it would be a fight between *greed* or feeling *too ashamed* to admit you were wrong.

Beginning with Louis Pasteur's same delusion, this kind of deception is going on with modern, conventional medicine to this day. It is hard to guess how much Pasteur's mind was eating away at itself, knowing he was receiving large sums of government money, but we're sure his mind was spinning. Let's look at the quote he said on his deathbed one more time. Remember it? - "The germ is nothing, the terrain is everything".

In our combined metaphors, our Rock Star Aaron would have finally concluded on his deathbed, "The raw brown sugar crystals are nothing...they are part of everything..."

With Aaron, think of the glass bowl as a cell membrane, the peanuts as cell parts, the raisins as other cell parts, and the raw brown sugar crystals as harmless viruses all around the cell. Pasteur was looking at raw brown sugar crystals in the wrinkles of raisins. All part of a normal cell! Pasteur must have finally realized that he was looking at harmless particles part of the whole. However, his mindset was based on the idea if something is too small to see, and he could convince people he sees something no one else does, he can blame disease on what nobody sees! He was so set on convincing the world that germs, bacteria, and viruses were making us sick he wouldn't admit he was wrong until right before he died.

Chapter 8
Where It All Shockingly Started

We now know "Tricky" Louis was keeping a lot of secrets. From the pages of Louis Pasteur's private notes, we find several revealing differences from what he actually told the public.[11] He did hundreds of experiments on rabbits, dogs, cows, silkworms, and sheep. His original success with Silkworm Blight gave him his initial popularity, but he considered the time he spent on the silkworms too excessive.

In 1881 he did an experiment on a flock of 60 sheep in Pouilly-le-Fort, France. According to the private notes, Pasteur was deceptive about the vaccine he injected in the experiment. His notes show he used a serum that *another* scientist had originally come up with. The lackluster outcome ended with several puzzled farmers wondering why so many sheep died after being told Pasteur knew what he was doing. The farmers were paid upfront for their sheep, but the deaths were kept secret from the public.[12]

In the fall of 1884, he makes notes about an experiment with 26 dogs that resulted in a 38% death rate. The small number of test subjects and that outcome give us numbers not very convincing to the science community. The deaths were kept secret.[13]

In the spring of 1885, he had four groups of ten dogs he did his rabies serum (vaccine) experiments on. The dogs would receive several shots spread apart day by day. Each shot would be successively more potent. He started his first experiment group of ten dogs on May 28th and the second group of ten soon after on June 3rd. In his notes, within 3 weeks after the second group was started, a few dogs died.

He pressed on and started his third group of ten dogs on June 25th, 1885, and the fourth group of ten on June 27th of the same year. After three weeks, once the fourth group was started, 20 of the 40 dogs had received their total amount of vaccines. After the 20 were given their last shot, guess how many of the 20 dogs died?? *Within 30 days* of the 20 dogs having had their final injection, ALL 20 OF THOSE DOGS WERE DEAD!! 20 OF HIS DOGS DIED!! [14] That's 50% DEAD. HIS DOG EXPERIMENTS WERE FAILURES!! Yet, he hid it from the world!! We are where we are today with medical fraud based on Louis Pasteur's deception. Half of the dogs DIED, and he still lied to everyone by saying his vaccines were a success!

Even more shocking, on June 22nd and 23rd, 1885, Pasteur and a doctor attended to an eleven-year-old girl. She had been bitten on the lip a full month before by her own puppy. The month passed, and a few days before Pasteur and the doctor saw her, she was complaining to her parents she had severe headaches. This was on June 20th and 21st, 1885, according to Pasteur's secret notes. Naturally, they took her to see a doctor. After Pasteur and the little girl's doctor examined her at the Hospital of St. Denis on June 22nd, 1885, they *"declared"* she had rabies. Pasteur and the doctor injected Pasteur's serum in her two times, once on that first afternoon and another right at midnight. Another tragedy! She *died* the second day at 10:30 am.[15] It's all in Pasteur's private notes. Pasteur hadn't even finished his dog experiments! He injected her between the 2nd and 3rd group of dog experiments. That innocent little girl's name was Julianne-Antoinette Poughon, an unfortunate victim of medical fraud and ego. We mention her name in remembrance of her short life and also all the other lives cut short since then because of one man's failed experimentations, which a corrupt system turned into *gospel truth.*

Not letting the death bother him, Pasteur and a doctor attended to young Joseph Meister, who had been bitten on the hand by an uncontrollable dog. They "declared" his symptoms to be rabies. He was given shots over a period of about two weeks. The shots started on July 6, 1885, *also before* Pasteur had finished his dog experiments.[16]

Because of Louis Pasteur's failed dog experiments, Julianne-Antoinette's death, and the unverified "success" in treating young Joseph Meister, he still flagrantly stated in his October 1885 paper:

"Fifty dogs of all ages and all races immune to rabies without a single failure." [17]

THE BIG LIE that started it all. Did you notice he exaggerated the number up to *50* dogs? [18]

Because of this "original sin" in science, modern medical institutions are continuously throwing darts in the form of sharp needles and barking up our trees with TV ads trying to convince us there is something wrong going on in our cells.

Our cells don't need assistance other than food, vitamins, oxygen, and water to stay alive. The narrative that cells get to a point where they are no longer recognizable as "self" comes from the idea that the body is going to attack itself. Conventional medicine calls it an auto-immune disease. In reality, science has proven time and time again that the innate intelligence of the body has the ability to break down, remove and/or repair cells. *CELLS COME AND GO; THEY KNOW EXACTLY WHAT THEY ARE DOING!* The dust on your dining room table comprises 20-50% dead skin cells. Did it hurt when the cells died? Did you even feel them fall off your skin? Every eight years, almost every cell in your body is a brand new cell, with the exception of the nervous system and the female reproductive eggs! Some cells regenerate within 24 hours.

Modern medical institutions teach Germ Theory as if it were a Gospel! In doing so, it keeps us in fear of things they claim to see under their microscopes that "could" kill us. It's false! Again, two words: IT'S FALSE! True, honest science has proven it's false. Germs serve a purpose that is helpful, and OUR CELLS KNOW *EXACTLY WHAT THEY ARE DOING!*

Many people say, "But what about pasteurization?" Aren't there harmful things in cow's milk? The only ones telling you that are the fearmongers.

Common sense would beg the question, "How did my grandparents ever stay alive after drinking raw milk?" The only benefit of pasteurization is the SHELF LIFE of milk! That's it. That is a convenience for the dairy industry. We can refer you back to Chapter 5. The fearmongers will tell you that the bacteria in milk is harmful and will give you food poisoning, miscarriages, kidney failure, and the list goes on. The massive dairy industry is pleased when we fear drinking raw milk.

Further on in history, interestingly enough, scientists decided randomly to alter the postulates a bit in 1937 so that *just maybe* they could prove experimentally that germs cause disease. Back in Koch's day, scientists only had the microscope (invented in the 1600s), so they couldn't see viruses yet. Eventually, in 1931 the electron microscope was invented, and some scientists thought they were seeing the "culprit virus" that they had blamed so many problems on. They are labeled "viruses", but we will explain later what scientists and virologist are now calling them in Chapter 21, now that we have a better picture and understanding of "viruses".

In 1937, Thomas Rivers came up with **Rivers' postulates.** These also make PERFECT sense and are logical.

They are as follows, now there are six:

1. The virus can be *isolated* from a diseased organism.

2. The virus can be *isolated* and made to grow in the cells of a new organism.

3. Proof of filterability—the virus can be separated from a medium that also contains bacteria.

4. The filtered virus will produce a comparable disease when the isolated virus is used to infect experimental animals.

5. The *virus can be re-isolated* from the infected experimental animal.

6. A specific immune response to the virus can be detected.[19]

So, did this help give researchers the proof they needed for blaming disease on bacteria or viruses? A big, fat NO! Nothing Further. NADA!

Researchers could not prove that a specific bacteria or virus causes ANY specific disease by using River's Postulates either! Try your best to find one.

There are many *paid* fact-checkers that claim on the internet that the researchers have met Koch's or River's postulates. It is doubtful that researchers even know what the postulates are when you read the procedures in the studies.

Dr. Tom Cowan, MD, states in the awesome book The Truth About Contagion (originally titled The Contagion Myth), *"No DISEASE attributed to bacteria or viruses has met all of Koch's postulates or all of River's criteria. This is NOT because the postulates are incorrect or obsolete (in fact, they are entirely logical)."* [20] You may ask, "What? How can that be?" **BECAUSE GERMS DON'T CAUSE DISEASE!!** But Big Pharma and all the organizations chasing profits will not let go of the Germ Theory fraud because it would be *way too costly.*

We need to change our paradigm and start BELIEVING that there is - "...No war going on between our cells in our bodies". Dr. Stefan Lanka – Freedom Talk 5 [21]

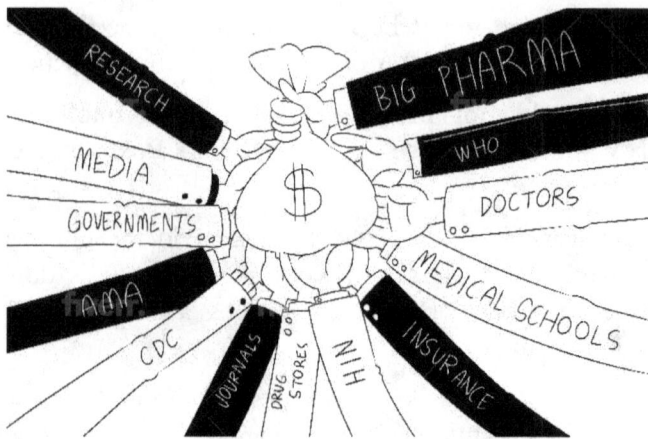

Chapter 9
Spider-Man vs Big Pharma and "The Snipes"

Let us make you scratch your brain. Do you like Spider-Man movies? Millions of people do. And millions of people know that most images in the movie are made with CGI (Computer Generated Imagery). However, when the movie is over, everyone knows that the movie was pure "make-believe". Right! Spider-Man doesn't exist in real life. Are we so conditioned to think anything we see on the internet or in the media is inherently real?

Certain virologists have used similar technology to claim they have isolated viruses. They use computer programs to find particles that *almost* fit together and then let computer programs fill in the empty holes. No DNA or RNA from any virus has ever been found. No virus has EVER been isolated! (More about this in Chapters 21 and 25).

The scientists that propose their findings with statements like "highly probable" and "most likely" are based on complete SPECULATION and ASSUMPTIONS. Deception is highly effective when one uses "smoke and mirrors". Have you ever heard a scientist in an authoritative position talk to the press with statements that sound like "word salad"? They haughtily ramble on and on.

Is it a coincidence that the images of the COVID-19 virus have the same colors as Spider-Man's suit?? Makes you go, hmmm...

Scientists around the globe know that to have proof-positive research, scientists present their findings, publish them, and then let other scientists peer-review the research to prove it *right or wrong*. Recall that word "reproducible".

Today we have "Science by Press Conference," as Robert F. Kennedy, Jr. wrote in his book "The Real Anthony Fauci," Bill Gates, Big Pharma, and the Global War on Democracy and Public Health.[22] You might recall Anthony Fauci in a quasi-press conference casually sitting on a sofa in the White House as he announced his *unverified* success with Remdesivir to treat COVID-19. Not so coincidentally, we also discovered he partially holds the patent on Remdesivir. Do you foresee a conflict of interest? If you had significant money to gain, would you promote something that has not been thoroughly tested? His findings were not published in any journal nor peer-reviewed for their effectiveness. That is ANTI-SCIENCE! Would you consider that *fraudulent?* Is it "smoke and mirrors"? Is he keeping secrets? There should be laws against this, don't you think? And yet, not a single word was spoken about better nutrition, building up immune systems, losing weight, getting plenty of Vitamin D, drinking clean water, reducing stress, etc. He was laser-focused on giving the public the ONLY OPTION of a VACCINE. It is as if someone should have given him a golden microphone. [23]

Narcissists love themselves and care little about anything or anyone else. Here's a question: Why hasn't Anthony Fauci written a book on his scientific findings? Search the internet! You won't find any. We can add, however, he has a pseudo-autobiography for sale. Do we need to say more? He has the same mindset as Louis Pasteur had? Or like Aaron, our Rock Star?

Even the coronavirus, "they say" (the CDC), has been supposedly isolated and studied, but where is the isolated virus? Why aren't the names of the researchers on the CDC's "special panels" that have found the virus revealed? Exactly who is coming to their "definitive conclusions"? Who is keeping secrets under the guise of "national security"? It is all crafty graphics and computer-generated pictures to *trick* the public into fearing and blaming a virus.

We know it's human nature not to want to feel like you have been deceived. Truth be told, it's a "hard pill to swallow" when we realize we have been deceived, pun intended. However, we are giving you the knowledge and power to start *THINKING FOR YOURSELF!*

The collective Big Pharma and medical government institutions remind us of a game called "Snipe Hunting". Do you know what a "Snipe" is? Young adolescents like the challenge of hunting for "Snipes" in the dark of night. You can picture young male adolescents holding a burlap sack and running as fast they can through trees and brush to catch as many "Snipes" as they can snag. The boys can't wait to *brag* about how many they caught the following day. Guess what?! The zinger is "Snipes" are fictitious creatures! You could hunt as many as you want and claim *more* than you bagged!

It sounds like what some virologists at the CDC have fed the public about viruses. It's time that we should stop falling for their deceptions. How many times will they cry wolf? Why should anyone believe the CDC when they are self-governed and self-regulated? They can say whatever they think is "highly probable" and "most likely" all they want with all the taxpayer money they receive, but why would you believe them?? Why *should* you believe them??

The virologists and scientists should look at man-made toxins from multiple sources, including the Wuhan lab and man-made genetic substances, the COVID-19 testing kits, the 5G testing, extreme *fear*, and the flu vaccines common to the people who were *diagnosed* with COVID-19. We'll get to those later.

One of the most comprehensive books written on the subject of viruses and the past fraud in the name of Big Pharma profits is **VIRUS MANIA: Avian Flu (H5N1), Cervical Cancer (HPV), SARS, BSE, Hepatitis C, AIDS, Polio...How the Medical Industry Continually Invents Epidemics, Making Billion-Dollar Profits at Our Expense by Torsten Engelbrecht, Dr. Claus Kohnlein, Dr. Samantha Bailey, MD, Dr. Stefano Scoglio, MD** [24]

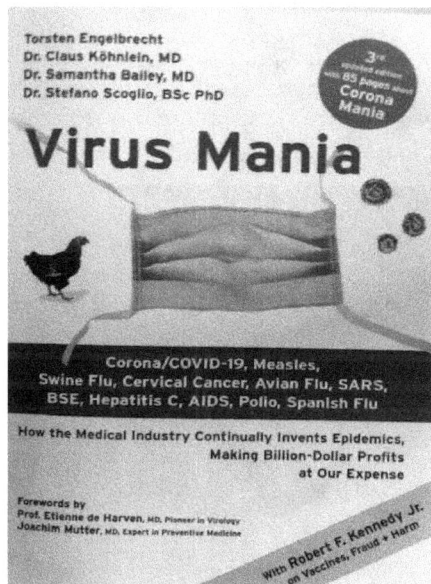

This book is a masterpiece of research and facts with over 2000 research articles. It's worth reading if you want *undeniable* certainty we have been duped!

Chapter 10
Spontaneous Generation?
Not to be mistaken for
Spontaneous Sex!

(just checking to see if you're still paying attention!)

So, what became of Bechamp's spontaneous generation theory? Oh, it still exists. It's been kept a big secret! But the truth will prevail!!

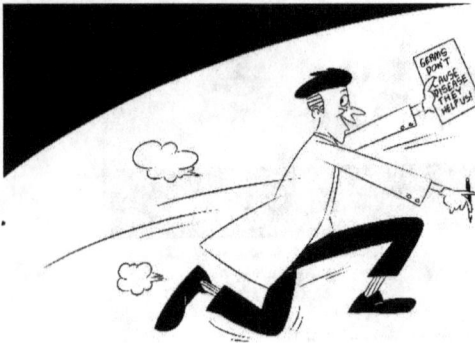

You are created with your own magical Divine power to heal! Bechamp proved that you have something called microzyma throughout your body. Microzyma sounds like something disgusting, so we like to call it Stardust. It's actually electromagnetic plasma (not to be mistaken for blood plasma) which is the same thing that makes up the stars and sun. No kidding! Stardust!!

Even Nikola Tesla, the great inventor, knew this back in 1920 when he wrote, "*All perceptible matter comes from a primary substance, or tenuity beyond conception, filling all space, the akasha or* **luminiferous ether,** *which is acted upon by the life-giving Prana or creative force (God), calling into existence in never-ending cycles all things and phenomena.*" -Nikola Tesla, Electric Body, Electric Health by Eileen Day McKusick.[25]

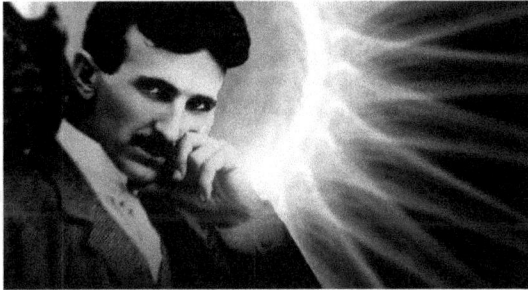

Your body is condensed electricity coming from Source (God) made from the ether!

"*The nitrogen in our DNA, the calcium in our teeth, the iron in our blood, the carbon in our apple pies were made in the interiors of collapsing stars. We are made of star stuff.*" -Carl Sagan (1934-1996) astrophysicist.

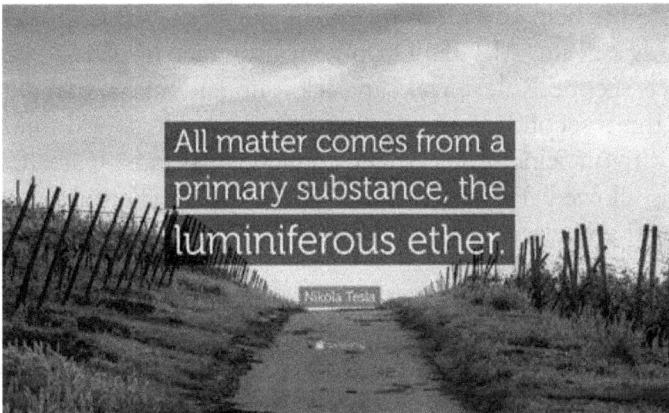

All matter comes from a primary substance, the luminiferous ether.

Nikola Tesla

So, follow us now...**Ether (light) is the ocean of luminosity** from which **ALL** originates. **Plasma** comes from the ether. **Plasma is** condensed light and sound energy waves that make up everything. And **Microzyma is your electric stuff present in you right now** to spontaneously generate **germs** like bacteria **to help you clean up garbage** and repair tissue in your body.

So, here's the order.:

1. You are made of ether (light) which condenses to…

2. Plasma which condenses to…

3. Your body cells and Microzyma (stardust), which transforms to…

4. *You guessed it: GERMS*…which are all part of you!

Germs break down *toxins, dead cells* and *dead cell debris* and *help repair* damage to keep you healthy. Remember, they are not the bad guys!

So, just to be clear…Louis Pasteur had *no proof* of the germ theory (it should be called the germ invention), which says that germs cause disease. Geisen showed us proof that Louis Pasteur falsified the results of his experiments.

Antione Bechamp proved germs (also known as microbes) *don't* cause disease. Germs help you clean up and repair tissue! The "Three Second Rule" is, once again, ALIVE! Drop your brownie? It's OK to go back to the "Three Second Rule". You can pick it up and take a BIG bite out of it within three seconds. Unless it happens on a picnic, no one likes the taste of dirt on icing! At least let your kids be kids again. Even four seconds is allowed. However, if you use a lot of chemical products to clean your floors, we advise caution!

Chapter 11
Microzymas or Stardust?

Bechamp concluded from his extensive research, "The micro-organisms known as 'disease germs' are thus either microzymas or their evolutionary bacterial form that are in or have proceeded from sick bodies (terrain)." These germs are there all the time! And these experiments have been repeated again and again.

Louis Pasteur's deathbed confession - *"The germ is nothing, the terrain [toxic tissue] is everything."* "Toxic tissues" are cells breaking down, cells between regenerating, cells damaged by foreign particles, cells that have been poisoned. Therefore, the cause of disease is damaged or sick tissue (terrain) not germs.

"Disease is born of us and in us." -Ethel Hume [26]

Like maids with sponges would be present to clean your house. You wouldn't blame the maid for the garbage! Also, picture germs breaking down a compost pile to dissolve it back to nature. We wouldn't call that an "infection." We would call that helpful!

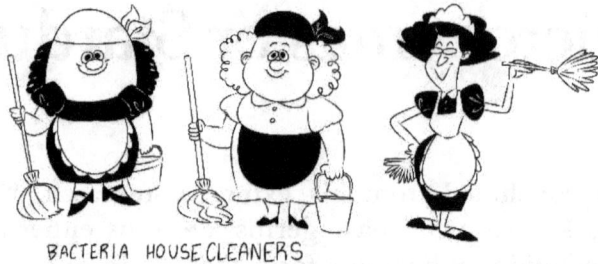

BACTERIA HOUSE CLEANERS

Two other comprehensive books that outline Pasteur's fraud are **Bechamp or Pasteur? A Lost Chapter in the History of Biology**, By Ethel Hume **1919** and **Pasteur: Plagiarist, Imposter; The Germ theory Exploded** by R.B. Pearson **1942**. They both declare their intentions openly: that *they wish to contribute to the undoing of a massive medical and scientific fraud.* [27] Note from the publisher of both books admin@adistantmirror.com.au 2017.

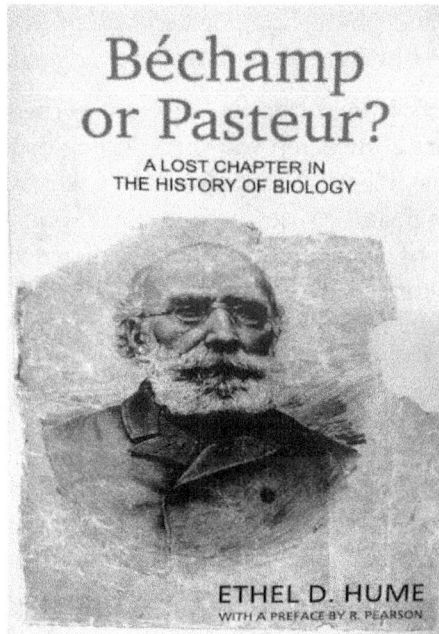

Béchamp
or Pasteur?

A LOST CHAPTER IN
THE HISTORY OF BIOLOGY

ETHEL D. HUME
WITH A PREFACE BY R. PEARSON

"Unthinking respect for authority is the greatest enemy of truth" - Albert Einstein.

---

150 years ago, the medical industry took off after using Louis Pasteur's false experiments and findings. They used propaganda to push the Germ Theory to make *trillions* of dollars on the sale of drugs and vaccines. They are still at it! How many prescription drug advertisements have you seen on TV within the last few days? It's modern-day propaganda. Big Pharma has media networks in the palm of its hand. It's a Catch-22 for the networks to either keep taking the advertisement money or find other ads and start honoring our health. Here's a suggestion, the next time you see a drug ad on TV, laugh and push the mute button! Did you know that the United States and New Zealand are the *only* two countries in the world that allow drug advertisements on TV? Big Pharma has been called out for taking a stock image of a baby being cradled by a

healthcare worker and photoshopping red bumps and scrapes onto the image claiming the baby has measles! More propaganda...

Our medical industry is based on the idea that germs make you sick. By now, we hope we are convincing you that nothing could be further from the truth. If you still have Semmelweis Reflexes, we will learn how germs, bacteria, fungi, and viruses *work together* in our cells. If you look at the dead cell tissue of a sick person under a microscope, you will *always* see germs *helping* clean up the area. And the cleanup and repair process *does* make you feel symptoms. "Think of it as a construction site, it's repairing itself." Caroline Markolin, PhD. Learninggnm.com. It's important to realize **YOUR SYMPTOMS ARE NOT YOUR SICKNESS.**

*SYMPTOMS ARE YOUR ALERT THAT YOU ARE **HEALING** OR **NEED REPAIR** either spiritually, emotionally, mentally, physically or a combination of all four!* Yes, the body can heal and protect itself.

Pearson wrote in 1942, "*The bacteria found in man and animals do not cause disease.* They have the same function as those found in the soil or in sewage or elsewhere in nature: they are there to rebuild dead or diseased tissues or rework body wastes, and *it is well known that they will not or cannot attack healthy tissues.* They are as important and necessary to human life as those found elsewhere in nature and are in reality just as harmless if we live correctly as Bechamp clearly showed." [28]

Bechamp was proving experimentally back in 1855 how germs come from microzyma (stardust) when the body needs to be cleaned up. The germs act like **house cleaners** produced from within the cells themselves when dying or threatened. Bacteria are electric generators when they're in the cell as mitochondria. When they come out of the cell, they act like maids or repairmen. Viruses (more accurately called exosomes, see Chapter 20) are in the cell as electric particles. And now we see, back in 2010, from the *atomic force microscope*, that they are released from the cell to act like sponges or cell phones. They are communication directors using cellular phones in your cells!

The immune system should actually be called the *support* system, made up of antibodies, anaerobic and aerobic bacteria, fungi, white blood cells, and viruses. You can now honestly think of them as "Good Guys".

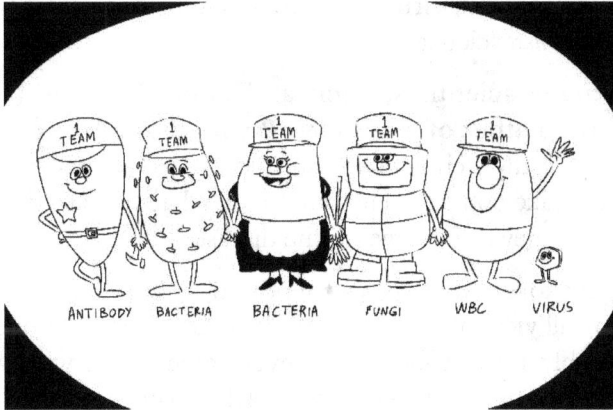

ANTIBODY   BACTERIA   BACTERIA   FUNGI   WBC   VIRUS

All living organisms, from the one-celled amoeba to your own body, are associations of these minute living electrical entities of microzymas. Bechamp, with the help of Professor Estor, found microzymas everywhere, in both healthy tissues and diseased. He proved that the microzymas were the basic units of life rather than the cell and were the builders of cell tissues. "They also concluded that bacteria are an evolutionary form of microzymas that occurs when a quantity of diseased tissues is broken up into its constituent elements." [29]

The germs of the air are merely microzymas, or bacteria, set free when their former habitat was broken up. Bechamp proved with several reproducible experiments that microzymas were the living remains of plant and animal life. In the recent or distant past, they were actually the primary *anatomical element* of that plant or animal studied.

He proved that on the death of an organ, its cells disappear, but microzymas remain imperishable. As the Bible talks about how we go from dust to dust,[30] the *dust* of the Bible, the *stardust* Carl Sagan writes about, and the *microzymas* of Bechamp's experiments are *all the same thing*!

Now we hope this is making sense. We realize when all you've ever been trained to think is that germs are bad, it's hard to wrap your head around the fact that they help us! We're trained to think of bacteria as either good or bad and that all viruses and fungi are bad. But that isn't what is reproduced in *honest* science.

There are many scientists, such as Rudolf Virchow (1821-1902), known as "the Father of Pathology," who drank bacterial cultures of so-called "deadly" cholera in front of his students to prove that bacteria don't make you sick. He said, "If live bacteria are transmitted to another person, they don't develop the disease."

Dr. Max Pettenkofer, M.D., is also reported to have swallowed cultures of cholera in full view of a class of students on more than one occasion. Yet, it is reliably reported that he never came down with any illness. How disgustingly brave, it takes the word "professionalism" to a new level!

Not to say that the disease "cholera" doesn't exist. It just isn't caused by a bacterium. The bacteria are there to help you clean out toxins and dead tissue when you have the disease.

That *none* of Louis Pasteur's experiments could be reproduced should make you consider the reason he got his nickname "Tricky" Louis. He made a lot of money and received a lot of fame for creating and repeating disinformation. Remember, he was, in a sense, lip-syncing into a golden microphone...

And now we have Big Pharma: the medical industry, the med schools, the CDC, the WHO, NIH, NIAID, Research Institutes, universities, the infectious disease industry, virologists, charitable foundations, private investors, etc. The list goes on and on for who profits *trillions* from this disinformation. The REAL disinformation! And remember that Big Pharma has a lot of the media by the "you-know-whats".

But just imagine...God, Higher Power, or whoever you consider as Source has equipped you with an electrical system that produces its own waste removal and repair system in the form of germs! Bechamp called this *spontaneous generation theory*. Although it is not a theory, it is a fact. A fact is something that can be proven.

If you garden or observe nature, you realize this happens in the soil. If you saw a dead animal in the forest covered by fly larva (which is one of nature's ways of decomposing a dead animal), you wouldn't say that the flies killed the deer.

If you saw a log decaying in the woods, you wouldn't blame the fungus. RIGHT!?!

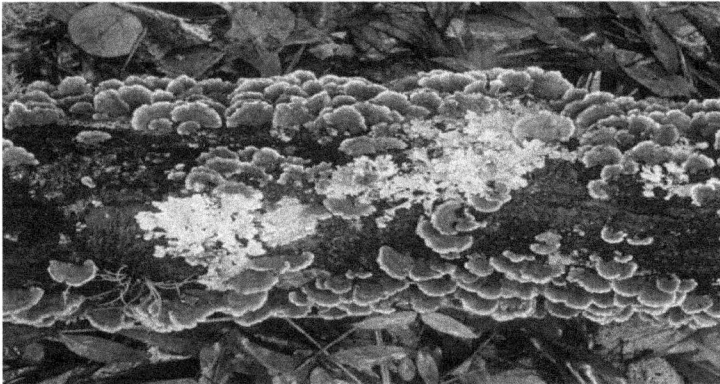

So, even though the germ theory (which states germs cause disease) is disproven by science, and Pasteur's experiments were revealed to be fraudulent, the medical industry is *still* teaching us all that we need to be *AFRAID* that germs will make us sick or even *KILL* us!

Here's a quote worth repeating that started off Chapter 4, **"If I could live my life over again, I would devote it to *proving* that germs *seek* their natural habitat, diseased tissue – rather than being the *cause* of the diseased tissue." -Rudolph Virchow (Father of Pathology).** [31]

"The specific disease doctrine is the grand refuge of _weak, uncultured, unstable minds_, such as now rule in the *medical profession*." -Florence Nightingale [32]

"The war on germs would seem to be (financially) a worthwhile one, most likely due to a mixture of human superstition and greed. Out of this war was born *the oppressive medical cartel* we are struggling with today. It's time we educate the people as to the truth and real purpose of these microbes and this fictional war. ***It's high time to say goodbye germ theory!*** **-Dr. William Trebing, Goodbye Germ Theory** [33] (More in chapter 38)

That you or I could breathe and cause grandma to die is as likely as a robber could murder you by giving you a hug and a kiss. There is *no scientific proof* that germs cause disease!

It's such a shocking revelation to realize you've been lied to. But we all have the choice to keep taking the red pill or to choose no pill. To be clear, taking the red pill is believing in the Germ Theory.

The advantage to waking up to the truth (taking no pill) is that you can truly realize your divine nature and power. Plus your self-healing capacity!

Your body is electromagnetic! It is full of trillions of chemical reactions, but they are coming from the *electric* source of light you are. **You are connected to the Divine Source, and all you need to do is improve your knowingness.**

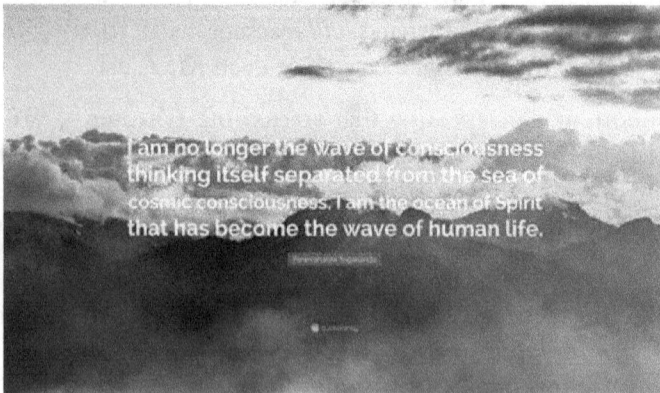

I am no longer the wave of consciousness thinking itself separated from the sea of cosmic consciousness. I am the ocean of Spirit that has become the wave of human life.

"I am no longer the wave of consciousness thinking itself separated from the sea of cosmic consciousness. I am the ocean of Spirit that has become the wave of human life."-Paramahansa Yogananda.

Chapter 12
Bacteria – Your house cleaners and repair service!

Your electromagnetic microzymas are what makes up your body. Bacteria are produced out of the microzymas when the body needs help cleaning up due to dead cells or repairs needed. Let's return to the original meaning of the word "germ". *Germ means new growth, to sprout up.* Seeds germinate! We all study that in grade school biology.

"It is widely accepted that mitochondria and plastids evolve from bacteria." [34]

Fortunately, when bacteria are unneeded for removing toxins or repair, they remain inside the cell as the mitochondria. They are the energy-producing electric batteries of your cells. **You have 4 times as many bacteria as you have cells (over 65 trillion) and you have trillions more variations of viruses!**

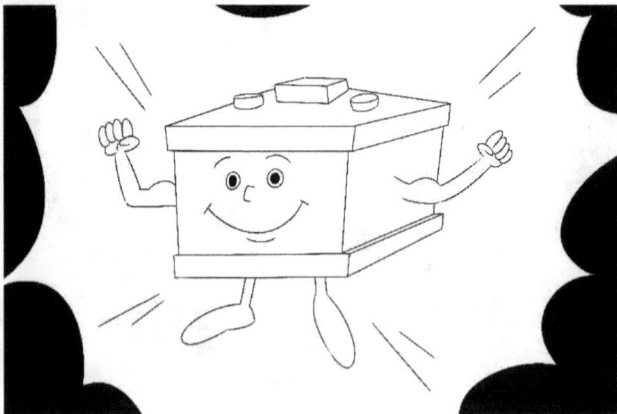

When bacteria are required by your body, they will change into a form needed to clean up toxins, dead cells, dead cell debris or repair. This is known as polymorphism. Staphylococcus bacteria are used in your skin and joints. Tuberculosis bacteria are used in your lungs and breast tissue. Streptococcus bacteria are used in your throat. To name a few. It might feel very strange to think that. But it's real! It's been proven, but Big Pharma doesn't want you to have the least bit of understanding about it. Not even an inkling! However, you will understand more as you read through the chapters coming up. Again, great decision to keep going!

Bacteria will secrete enzymes to break down your damaged tissue. Waste products of the bacteria excretions or bacterial "poop" cause some irritation which causes inflammation. **Inflammation is needed to dilate the blood vessels and bring more blood to the area to help remove the waste products. Yes, inflammation is part of the whole picture!**

Inflammation of this type is *assisting* your body by having more blood in an area that will help remove the damaged tissue. Bacteria need to do their work in a fluid, warm and acidic environment. However, doctors call this an infection. You aren't being infected; you are being repaired. Again, that may sound completely backwards. It goes against everything we've ever heard in our lives. Resist your Semmelweis Reflex! We'll bet you have already washed your hands several times today. When you realize that you could wash your hands 100 times in one day and that there would still be harmless germs and bacteria on your hands, you will relax! If we all think that way, one by one our collective consciousness will let go of the Germ Theory and the *fear* it gives us!

Chapter 13
Is an infection bad?

When you have damaged or dead tissue due to toxins, bacteria will be produced to help you remove it from the body. Excretions of bacteria will often create symptoms called an infection. Do you see why any time you have an infection, bacteria will be present? The infection is helping you remove dead tissue and toxins.

Florence Nightingale, the famous nurse, said, "True nursing *ignores* infection, except to prevent it. Cleanliness and fresh air from open windows, with unremitting attention to the patient, are the only defense a true nurse needs." [35]

These excretions of the bacteria (infection), which are often pus and fluid, will accelerate the removal of the waste products and speed up the healing.

If you use antibiotics, which kill the bacteria, you will stop or slow down the healing process from occurring. You will also damage the mitochondria in your cells made of bacteria. The symptoms might improve, but *then you still have the buildup of damaged tissue or toxins to remove.* That buildup of damaged tissue will result in more "diseased" tissue, which can sometimes lead to a large overgrowth which conventional medicine would mislabel "a tumor". During the body's healing phase, the so-called "tumor" will start to be broken down and removed from the body by bacteria. By *what* bacteria are still left! Are you still having Semmelweis Reflexes? The tumor will encapsulate if your body doesn't have enough bacteria due to the overuse of *antibiotics!* Did that sound strange?? We bet it did! Semmelweis again. If the encapsulated tissue growth (tumor) is pressing on your superior vena cava, then yes, you should have it surgically removed! The surgery would make sense because the superior vena cava is the large vein that returns blood back to the heart.

Here's another example, if you were dealing with a chronic throat infection, most doctors will think it's *caused* by streptococcus bacteria. Yet streptococcus bacteria are there in your throat *all the time*! You will get treated with an antibiotic, which will kill your "bacterial maid service" of streptococcus bacteria on the tonsils. Doctors might assume the tonsils are far too full of garbage (dead cells or toxins) to heal on their own. Your doctor may eventually say you need to have a tonsillectomy due to all the dead cell buildup. When we fall and scrape our knee, we soon get a dry, brown-colored scab. When dealing with the tonsils, the ugly-looking yellow patches are simply an *internal scab*. When babies get thrush, it's simply the inside of the mouth and tonsils scabbing over and repairing. The cells are healing.

A much better plan would be to remove the stress or physical toxins that had caused the dilemma in the first place. Then the bacteria would not need to clean up any of the dead cells, and your symptoms and scabs will go away for good. Take a minute to recall the last time you had a scab. Scabs are unpleasant to look at, but when has anyone seen a scab overgrow and take over a whole body and cause death?? Some "cancer" growths are simply *internal scabs* repairing cell overgrowth.

Stay tuned, keep reading! Things will come together!

From Dr. William Trebing's 25 years of clinical research, he says, "When your body has reached a certain level of toxicity from your external environment, or more likely your dietary and drinking habits, what does the medical establishment say to do once they detect these bacterial healing agents? Wipe them out with antibiotics (translates: "against-life") and other types of drugs, and further turn your internal body fluids into a *toxic* soup."- Dr. Trebing [36]

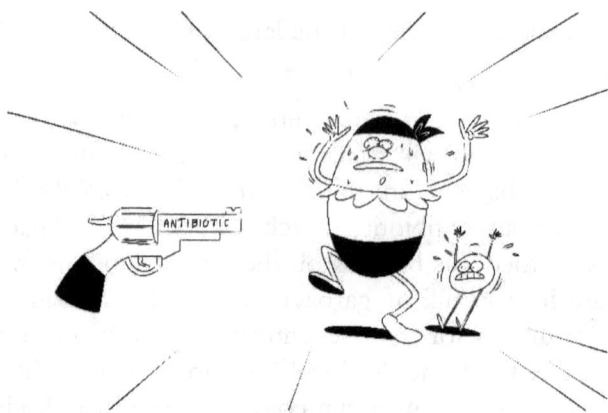

To be clear, you have been erroneously told that germs cause disease. The truth is every bacteria and virus you have been told cause disease can exist *harmlessly* inside you! Cholera, staphylococcus, tuberculosis, Ebola, streptococcus, E. coli are all in your body, ready to be made from the microzymas when you need them. When you are healthy, you don't need as many bacteria or germs for cleanup or repair.

When you are sick or toxic, germs will show up (because they are produced by your body out of the microzyma) and cause symptoms of inflammation or infection which are there to clean up the actual problem.

The problem isn't the infection. The infection results from toxins. Focus on the toxins! Do you have any emotional, spiritual, mental, or physical toxins that are active or present? Clean up the toxins and resolve any life conflicts to help the germs do their job, and your infectious symptoms will go away.

As we pointed out before, sometimes medical intervention *is needed*. Sometimes, you need medical intervention to *slow down* the infectious repair if the symptoms are painful or life-threatening. Our common sense would know in extreme situations when emergency intervention is needed. Lumpectomy and cataract surgery are good examples of the amazing advancement of medical technology. And yes, you can trust your intuition instead of listening to Drug Ads! Keep reading! This could save your life or the life of someone you know.

This diagram of the life cycle of a bacterium depicts how bacteria are "born" spontaneously out of the microzyma into somatids and then further transfer into other life forms. This all takes place within your own body.

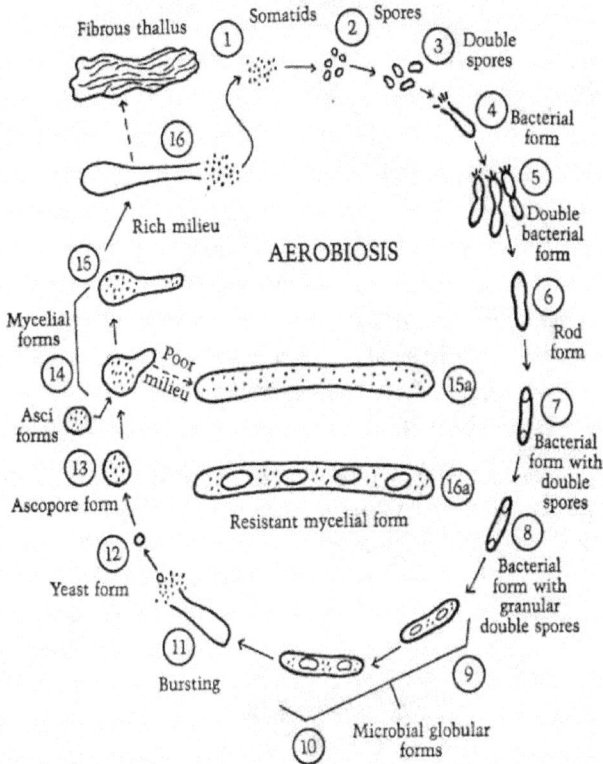

Fibrous thallus
Somatids 1 2 Spores
3 Double spores
16
4 Bacterial form
Rich milieu
15 5 Double bacterial form
AEROBIOSIS
Mycelial forms
6 Rod form
14
Poor milieu
15a
7
Asci forms
13
16a
Bacterial form with double spores
Ascopore form
Resistant mycelial form
8 Bacterial form with granular double spores
12
Yeast form
11
Bursting
9
10 Microbial globular forms

Here's an excerpt from Rational Bacteriology by doctors Verner, Weint, and Watkins. *"Extensive studies of bacteria show definitely that there are no fixed species. A coccus can become a bacillus, a spirili, and vice versa. Streptococci and pneumococci interchange. All bacteria either acquire or lose virulence depending upon their environment. Bacteria change to molds and vice versa in response to adequate environmental stimuli. Furthermore, they can resolve into their smallest form, (somatids, sporatids and microzyma)."* [37]

Every time you eat yogurt or drink kombucha, you are taking in LOTS of anaerobic bacteria that are just part of the fermentation process. GOOD and BAD BACTERIA are inaccurate names. They are misnomers. Bacteria are part of the terrain, part of everything. The terrain makes us think of trail mix with jellybeans and wrinkled raisins! It ALL goes together.

Bacteria can also biodegrade many pollutants, such as heavy metals. It's been proven!

E. coli bacteria are regarded as a major cause of food poisoning, but it's also widely recognized that E. coli normally reside in the intestines of healthy people. *"The fact that they are found in healthy people who do not suffer from food poisoning is a situation that fails to meet Koch's First Postulate, which means that E. coli cannot be the cause of any disease including food poisoning!"*- 1998 article entitled, "Physical Properties and Heavy-metal Uptake of Encapsulated Escherichia Coli Expressing a Metal Binding Gene," from **What Really Makes You Ill**.

As the amazing book **Goodbye Germ Theory** puts it emphatically, ***"BACTERIA ACTUALLY BOOST IMMUNITY AND AID IN THE HEALING PROCESS!"*** [38]

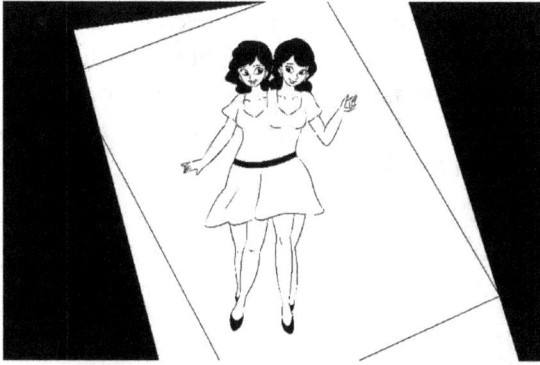

Chapter 14
The Story of Masha and Dasha

Picture this sad story about conjoined twins Masha and Dasha. Their new mother was told that they had died at birth. However, the truth was that they were sent to be studied at an institute near Moscow.

Because they shared the same blood, they should've experienced all the childhood diseases like measles, flu, and colds at the same time one of the two got sick. However, it was seen repeatedly that these diseases were experienced by each one of them at different times. Why is this so? Why did one become ill with a childhood disease, like measles, for example, while the other did not? The measles "bug" was assumed to be in both of their bodies, in their collective bloodstream. So why didn't they both get measles? Because measles is NOT *caused* by a virus or germ, and neither is the flu or cold! We'll cover more on those in Chapter 17 and 18.

Dr. Ryke Hamer, MD, proves in his work called, The Five Biological Laws, that germs don't cause disease but instead *play a vital role during the healing phase.* Dr. Hamer, MD concluded about germs after 30 years of research, *"They live in harmony with all organisms of the ecological milieu in which they have developed over millions of years."* [39]

Chapter 15
What about Fungi?

Fungi also evolve from microzymas. The life cycle of germs in the diagram of a bacteria actually involves fungi if they are needed for cleanup or repair, as in many cancers.

Fungi are like house cleaners or repairmen with hazmat suits. When an area of your body has been toxic for a longer time, fungi often polymorph from bacteria to help break down the dead cells.

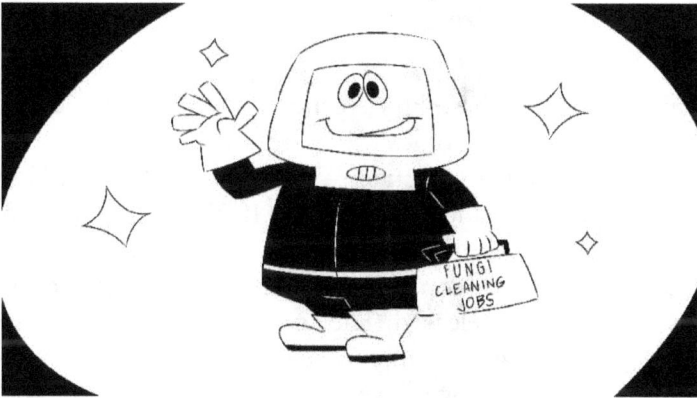

Fungi like candida remove certain types of cancer like breast cancer, pancreatic cancer, lung cancer, and colon cancer, along with other cellular debris in the healing phase. Remember the picture of the dead log with all the Fungi growing on it? It's in its breakdown phase!

Chapter 16
So, what's the truth about viruses?

So, what actually is a virus? **This is where it gets really exciting!** Well, we hope exciting isn't an overstatement for you, but at least you'll *see the truth of how God made you so AMAZING!*

To understand this, you REALLY need to open up your mind to the fact that your awesome, amazing body is always trying to help you stay healthy and remove toxins.

For example, you have these little, teeny tiny particles called viruses or, more recently called, "exosomes" that are made in all your cells to be released when the cell is threatened. When released, they act like electric sponges, garbage bags, and cell phones. If there is something toxic around the cell, it will release these particles so the cell can be protected. These little particles also communicate with all the other cells of the body once they've been released. They communicate there is something harmful present and that it is time to get to work! Do you know the big orange cones and barrels we have a love-hate relationship with when we're driving through construction zones? Exosomes put miniature orange cones and barrels up inside our bodies. Such hard-working and intelligent sugar crystals!

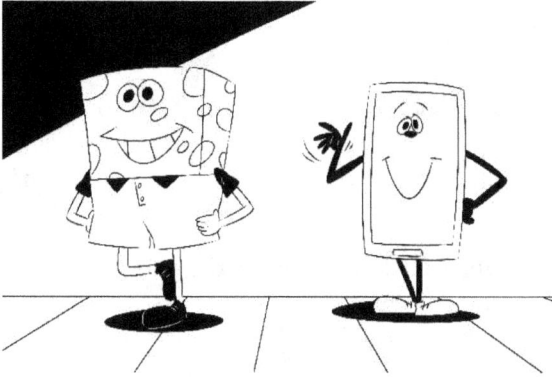

Viruses (including the coronavirus) are about 20-400 nm (10x smaller than a bacteria). They are the most abundant biological entities on the planet. There are 380,000,000,000,000 (380 trillion) viruses *in you*. Good thing they AREN'T actually BAD!

You immediately asked in your head, "But, Doc, COVID-19 killed so many people, right?!?" We'll help you understand that complex issue better in Chapter 23.

Viruses contain either an mRNA or a DNA strand, and it's surrounded by a protein shell. What does that mean? It means they exist within the cell as nano-particulates. All scientists have agreed that viruses are non-living. Some scientists say it's only cellular debris. However, scientists who look can see that they are very geometrically shaped. *They are far too beautifully shaped to be garbage.*

Most scientists have been claiming that viruses cause disease by invading the cell, multiplying and "infecting" it. This unfortunate *reversal* of the truth has created an untold loss of health and life. Because viruses don't ever "invade" or infect a cell! They help you!! Did the Semmelweis Reflex rear its head?

And guess what? Viruses can't move because they are NOT alive!! Yes! Viruses are NOT alive. They don't travel around in your spit when you cough. Consider the virus as the most numerous form on earth. As we already mentioned, viruses are actually helpful in sustaining the biological processes on the planet rather than infecting everyone and everything.

Is Hand Sanitizer sounding a little ironic yet? Please, yes, wash your hands to be clean from dirt and grease. Obviously, as a human species, we can't resist eating French fries with anything other than our fingers. Germs and viruses are simply part of the terrain!

Most current scientists look at germs as dangerous without ever looking at the actual research (which is nowhere to be found for infectious disease)! Everyone was told somewhere in our schooling that germs are infectious, and we never looked at the scientific evidence. We encourage you to research for yourself. It's all in plain sight that the reverse is the truth. We are on a mission to get more people to question the Germ Theory!

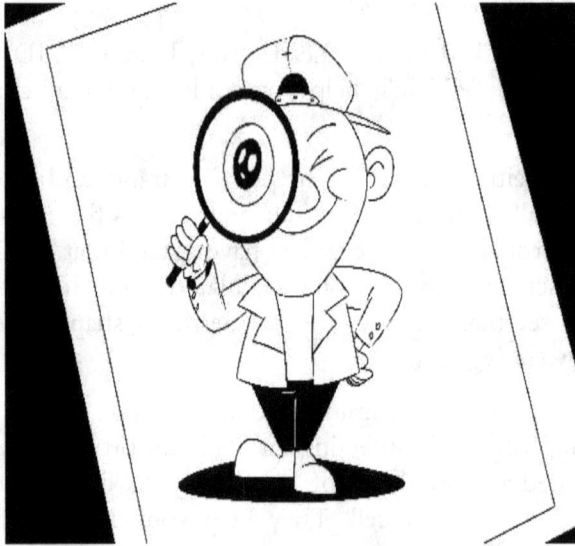

The truth is viruses are only *released by the cell* when threatened *to protect the cell* or to communicate with other cells. *They will be present when there is any disease process because they are assisting.* They are supporting you anytime they are present! But this truth does not fit into the "virus causes disease" agenda. And that

agenda leads us to a MASS DECEPTION started and continued today by Big Pharma, conventional medicine, and government science organizations worldwide. Think of viruses as sugar crystals in the wrinkles of raisins. Harmlessly coexisting!

We realize we keep hitting the same point. But everywhere you read, unless you research, you will find the same misinformation about germs. If you re-think this one well-kept secret, you'll do a lot for your own health!

There are about 1 million viruses that would fit on a pencil tip. Your body is *filled* with them. There are over 10 *billion* species of viruses in one gallon of seawater. *If* they were truly deadly or dangerous, you really shouldn't go in the ocean water! And, if Big Pharma or the CDC could convince you that seawater was dangerous so they could sell you an anti-viral body condom, they would! At the very least, they would *own the patent*. But viruses aren't deadly or dangerous. **They simply help you when you need it.** Because God made you amazing!! Once again, they come out of the electromagnetic microzyma or Stardust (as we like to think of it) to help you live toxin free and have intracellular communication.

Because, honestly, we are completely and utterly filled with viruses, it ISN'T even logical that they are evil, infectious particles. Yes, the computer "virus" infects your computer and messes with your information, but you are not your computer! You CANNOT be hacked!! Your common sense can be hacked by the media and pharmaceutical companies that sell vaccines. But that is about it. Together we can put an end to the MASS DECEPTION!

Remember the quote in Chapter 2 - "The bigger the lie, the more people will believe it."

Let's look at colds and influenzas.

Chapter 17
What about contagion? It seems like people catch a cold or the flu.

In our 30 years of clinical practice, we never worried about "catching" a cold or the flu. We've had well over 270,000 patient visits and always thought that if our immune systems stayed healthy, it wouldn't matter what was flying around. And we rarely got sick. After doing research, we realize it was NOT about our immune systems and germs.

There are never any disease-causing germs flying around in a person's spit as we are trained to imagine. Yes, it's great *not* to get sneezed or coughed on, but *real* studies have proven you *can't* get sick that way or make anyone else sick that way! And there is NO study you will find that proves contagion if you do your research. Which you should!

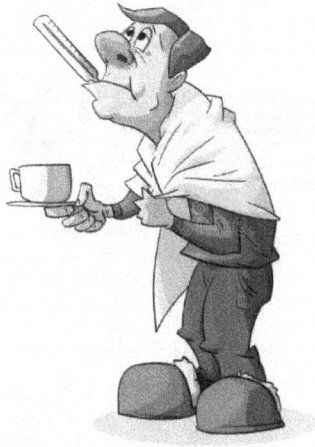

Flus and colds are the way your body releases toxic buildup or resolves a life-mental conflict. Usually, we have more toxins of stress, chemicals, food, alcohol during the holidays or "flu season," so it's common for people to "catch a cold or the flu" at that time. We are not catching anything from someone else…We are *reacting psychological and biologically in the same way as those close to us are.* We actually can "catch" the fear of getting sick because someone around us is ill. Or we can experience the same conflicts as others from the mere image of seeing them sick.

Chapter 18
Flus and Colds
Explained More

Dr. Ryke Hamer MD states, "Contrary to the common belief, (colds and flu) are not at all related to viruses (which have never been scientifically proven) but rather to an *"indigestible morsel conflict"* and *"territorial anger conflict"* experienced simultaneously by a group of people (city residents, villagers, family members, colleagues, schoolmates, roommates, friends) who share the same anger-environment (at home, at work, in daycare, in kindergarten, at school, in nursing homes, etc.). At first, the word "morsel" probably sounds odd, but it really is the right word to use because it can refer to any small piece or thing. The morsel could be physical or psychological. Dr. Hamer has thousands of case studies that prove this and are reproducible. His work, called German New Medicine, keeps getting suppressed by Big Pharma and others. He discovered humans and animals have Five Biological Laws that govern disease processes. He mapped out these diseases by reading CT (Computerized Tomography) brain scans of all his patients. Of the 6,500 cases of cancer patients he had, 90% were still alive after 10 years! That's far above Conventional Medicine statistics.

Think about it; children are sent off to their first daycare experience. Many come down with a "cold" or sickness several days or weeks after they start. Many experience a new conflict and get triggered by the new environment that is not their familiar home, the separation from their parent, and meeting strange new faces. Once they *get over their conflict,* they cough, sneeze and blow their noses because their bodies are breaking down the small cell over-growths. We attribute this to "catching germs" and something must be "going around." The children are, in reality, experiencing the same *"territorial conflict"* or possibly a *"stink conflict"* (yes, we call it a "stink conflict!" Semmelweis, anyone?) The life-mental conflict triggers the psyche-brain-organ to run a Special Biological Program (SBP) as German New Medicine defines it. It's a simple cold! If the shock is bigger for one child than another, it could trigger what conventional medicine would label an upper respiratory infection or the FLU! Especially if the child has a difficult time resolving the conflict promptly.

"Territorial anger conflicts can involve large numbers of people. Unexpected, upsetting political decisions, for example, can trigger regional conflict shocks followed by a "stomach flu" outbreak in the affected population after the conflict has been resolved. Stomach Flu epidemics typically occur after natural disasters such as floods or earthquakes, during the resolution phase." www.learninggnm.com [40]

We've all seen flocks of birds flying in spectacular shapes in the sky. Sea creatures swim in pods. When was the last time you watched the dolphins swimming in the ocean? We, as humans, are creatures that behave the same way here on the ground! We can all face a conflict and react together, simultaneously on our psyche-brain-organ. We go through a life-mental conflict, and we all get scared by it; most of us never realize what "hits" us. We go through what we erroneously believe is a pandemic blamed on a non-proven virus. The government agencies know they can coerce us using psychology against us! Now, are you seeing why so many people are shouting fraud about the pandemic?

Can that be true? We are trained our whole life to stay away from sick people so we don't get sick. Or we need to stay home when we're sick, so we don't pass anything along. But real, honest science does not support that. Much of what we do is based on propaganda to *perpetuate the Germ Theory*. Especially to perpetuate selling drugs and vaccines. And who funds the propaganda? Those who make money on drugs and vaccine sales. Follow the money, my friend!

A study was done in February of 1921 by the *Hygienic Laboratory #123* of the US government. (Another disgustingly brave experiment). The study was done where they tried to contaminate 62 Navy personnel with the flu in every possible way. They took sputum from influenza cases and sprayed it down their throats and on their foods. They kept the Navy personnel in constant contact with flu patients. The conclusion of the study showed **"no appreciable reactions."** *Nothing* showed that the subjects of the experiment caught anything from anyone! [41]

We are trained to believe that a cold "virus" is transmitted through your spit or mucus particles when you cough, sneeze or just breathe. The particles are thought to be inhaled by another person, who then becomes infected by the virus, which travels through their body to the affected part of the lung tissue. The transmission of viral particles has never, ever been observed or proven! Viral particles are only ever observed in a lab under an electron microscope. And even then, it is difficult to see viruses due to their tiny size. *The transmission of viruses in the air is only an _assumption,_ as is their ability to travel through a human body!*

Remember, germs, bacteria, and fungi are not the bad guys! We can add viruses to the list!

A very thorough analysis of all diseases can be found in Dr. Hamer's work.

We strongly encourage you to visit the websites

www.gnmonlineseminars.com

and www.learninggnm.com

for an in-depth look at German New Medicine (GNM) and any diagnosis you are curious about, from cancers to canker sores!

Chapter 19
Exosomes are Viruses?

Dr. Andrew Kaufman, MD, is a well-known researcher of viruses and exosomes. He has a great question-and-answer website we would highly recommend! [42]

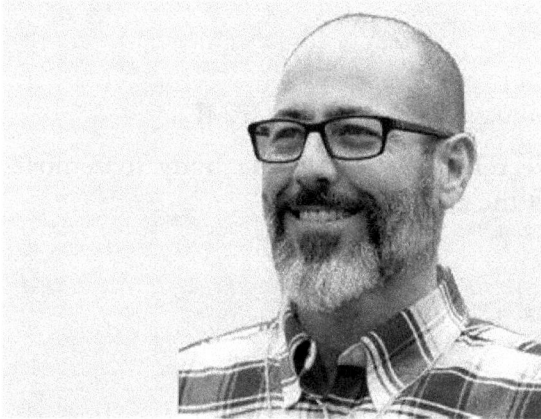

andrew@andrewkaufmanmd.com

When we were first doing our research about viruses, we came across a YouTube video by Dr. Andrew Kaufman, MD, in early 2020. He was being interviewed about COVID-19, and he mentioned how he thought viruses were **exosomes** that had been recently discovered. His first explanations started our quest to discover the truth. Big Pharma didn't squash **exosome** research because they didn't realize these scientists were researching viruses. Any **exosome (virus) research negates germ theory and vaccines.** And now we have a lot of it! Remember, you can think of viruses/exosomes as the guys with miniature walkie-talkies who put up tiny orange road construction cones and barrels inside your cells!

According to James Hildreth, MD, President and Chief Executive Officer of Maharry Medical College, a former professor at John Hopkins and HIV researcher, "The *virus is fully an* **exosome** *in every sense of the word.*" **Exosomes are released when the cells are** *in the presence* **of:**

- Toxic substances

- Stress (fear)

- Ionizing radiation

- Injury

- Electro-magnetic frequencies (EMF)

Exosomes are released to help the body to remove these toxins and to protect the cell!

Chapter 20
What Are Live Cell Studies Versus Dead Cell Studies?

In 2010, the Atomic Force Microscope was used to view *live* cells in relation to the viruses (exosomes) by Shivana Sharma, who has a PhD in Biomedical Engineering. She was observing how these particles come out of the cells to *aid* the cell. And the research shows that exosomes and viruses are the exact same thing!

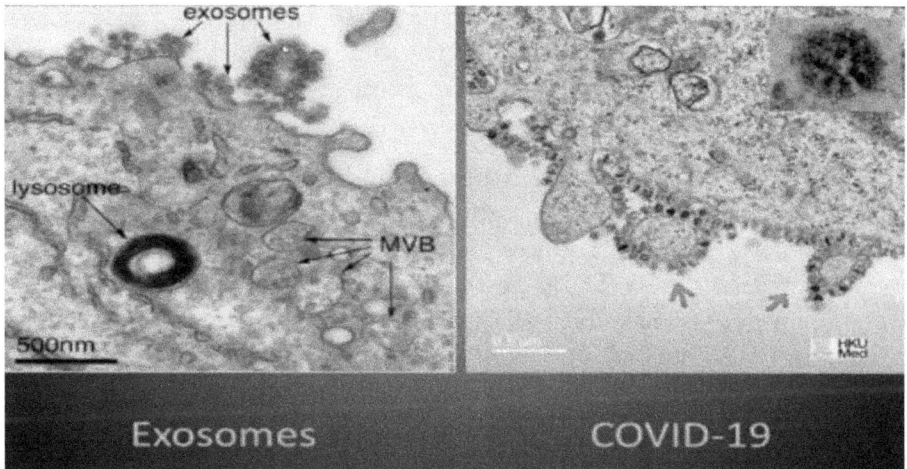

Exosomes   COVID-19

"Exosomes (viruses) act much like a sponge preventing the toxins for a time from attacking the cell while toxins that are not corralled are left to burrow through cell membranes," says another study by a co-senior investigator, Ken Caldwell, PhD. [43]

Another researcher, Dr. Ian Dixon, writes, "The more research that is done into exosome function, the more we discover the pivotal role they play in development, in maintaining health, in the processes of aging and in disease." He also states, "Exosomes have been shown to be key mediators of cell-to-cell communication, delivering a distinct cargo of lipids, proteins, and nucleic acids that reflects their cell of origin. Exosomes released by regenerative cells such as stem cells, for example, are potent drivers of healing and repair." [44]

They can see these exosomes (viruses) are actually surrounding the toxins like garbage bags or sponges and communicating with other cells to alert the cells to toxins.

Once you realize the research that viruses are coming out of your cells to help you and that there is NO research showing the virus causes any disease (including the coronavirus), you will have a mind that is at ease! Viruses, germs, bacteria and all microbes are present all the time and only get released when you have some kind of toxin present (stress, previous vaccines, 5-G, testing chemicals on swabs). They get released NOT to make you sick but to help you cleanse and get healthy. You will never fear them! You will welcome them!! You are literally filled with viruses, and you are not *scared of yourself.*

We are *all* trained by Big Pharma propaganda. ALL of Big Pharma make their living by keeping the same story alive about germs, bacteria, viruses, cancers, drugs and vaccines. Remember the Spider-Man-colored CGI images of COVID-19? We hope, by now, you will *LAUGH* at the scary image. It's make-believe! We can hear Batman say to Robin, "It's only an Exosome. Let's get out of here and fight a real crime!"

Yes, you will see viruses when you study the discharge of sick people BECAUSE VIRUSES (AND BACTERIA) WILL BE THERE TO HELP REMOVE THE TOXINS AND HELP REPAIR OR REMOVE UN-NEEDED CELLS. The only thing they have ever used to look at viruses are electron microscope pictures of non-moving virus particulates combined with other particulates from dead animal tissue. When the atomic force microscope was invented in 1989, from then on, we saw all kinds of positive research on exosomes (viruses).

It's really the perfect system that mother Nature (God) came up with for our planet to be self-cleaning and self-healing! That very few understand how Mother Nature works in our bodies is a testament to the deceiving propaganda of Big Pharma. They have taught every doctor, teacher, and parent to repeat the same Germ Theory that Louis Pasteur preached back in the 1860s *with no proof whatsoever.* Oh, they may have a few studies that they PAID researchers for, but if they are asked for proof that they EVER isolated a virus, THERE IS NONE! Despite all the court-documented requests for evidence, a virus has never been isolated!! Keep reading!

Chapter 21
Has a Measles Virus ever been isolated?

Dr. Stefan Lanka offered $100,000 to anyone in Germany who produced genuine scientific proof of the *measles virus*. In 2016 the courts in Germany found *no one provided any of the necessary proof of a measles virus*. Seriously? We all know there's a measles virus, right? Wrong! It's never been isolated and injected in a healthy person and caused measles...EVER! There's a skin condition called measles. But it's NOT caused by a virus. It's a skin condition that derives from a separation conflict and runs its course through a conflict phase and a healing phase (repair phase) of a Significant Biological Program (SBP) as defined in German New Medicine and the Five Biological Laws of Nature as discovered by Dr. Ryke Gerd Hamer. The red bumps we see are visible symptoms of the body healing its own skin. The same applies to Monkey Pox! Ever wonder why they say Monkey Pox lasts between 4 to 6 weeks?? The media stories and pictures are fear-mongering by our governments and institutions, and THAT drives us to comply to their demands and keep us in fear!

The original term "smallpox" was a label given to anyone in previous centuries that presented with any form of rash on the skin. Today, smallpox is labeled measles, chickenpox, or monkeypox.

"What we today call chickenpox, monkeypox, scarlet fever, measles, rubella, tanapox, herpes zoster, erythema multiforme, molluscum contagiosum, impetigo, dermatitis, and so on were labels that were created to separate the previously unified term "smallpox" for conditions accompanied by a rash." - Ekaterina Sugak, Naturalpath www.ekaterinasugak.com

The coronavirus is a perfect example of a virus viewed as a culprit but never isolated! Even the head of the Chinese CDC said when he was asked by NBC Nightly News why they didn't share information with the US regarding the coronavirus and its threat to public health. Dr. Wu Zunyou said, **"They didn't isolate the virus, that's the problem."** [45] And why not? *Because the virus isn't the cause of anything, and they can't isolate it and prove that it is*!! If you study the research, it is computer-generated pictures in fancy words. It's the trickery of CGI and a scary "you could die" diagnosis that literally scares the "breath out of us" along with ulterior motives to sell the public on drugs and vaccines. The diagnosis *itself* is a biological shock/conflict, and innocent people unknowingly start down the path of a Significant Biological Program (SBP). Whether the coronavirus had ever been isolated has been challenged in court many times, and each time the ruling states that the coronavirus has NEVER been isolated!

We get this seems crazy. We mean could scientists REALLY have NO PROOF of viruses causing any disease? Remember the postulates meant to be used to diagnose an infectious disease? That is the scientific method, and *not one virus has been isolated to show it causes disease!*

Have you ever heard of anyone being tested to see whether their breath contained the coronavirus? No, even the swabs can't test for a virus. They test for an antibody, which will be present in the case of *any* toxin. Even the inventor of the PCR test, Kary Mullis (who mysteriously died in 2019), was quoted as saying you *can't* use his test to diagnosis anything!

Let's look at who Kary Mullis was.

Chapter 22
The Kary Connection and
ADJUSTABLE PCR Tests

Dr. Kary Mullis (1944-2019) won the Nobel Prize in Chemistry in 1993. He was another brilliant scientist. Mullis, for years, was one of Dr. Fauci's biggest critics. Mullis said, "Guys like Fauci get up there and start talking and you know he doesn't know anything really about anything, and I'd say that to his face. Nothing. The man thinks you can take a blood sample and stick it in an electron microscope and if it's got a virus in there, you'll know it... He doesn't understand electron microscopy and he doesn't understand medicine. And he should not be in the position he is in..." [46]

It could be phrased that Kary Mullis "conveniently" died in August of 2019, two months before the EVENT 201 was rehearsed by Bill Gates, Anthony Fauci, et al., and right before the pandemic was announced. His official cause of death was "labeled" pneumonia, but several scientists and professionals question it. EVENT 201 was a "dress rehearsal" in the case that a pandemic broke out around the world. It included "...techniques for controlling official narratives, silencing dissent, forcibly masking large populations, and leveraging the pandemic to promote mandatory mass vaccinations." Now you know why people have been saying "Plandemic"! Operation Warp Speed had "vast military involvement" that included 21 civilian health leaders *outnumbered* by 61 military personnel that included four Generals. Dress rehearsals have always taken place before any announcement of a virus! The movie "War Games" is similar. You most likely have never heard of Dark Winter 2001? Atlantic Storm 2003? Global Mercury 2003? Lockstep Simulation 2010? SPARS 2017? Crimson Contagion 2019? You can research them more in the bibliography notes or on the internet using a non-censoring search engine like DuckDuckGo.com because you will find little about it using Google. [47]

"Scientists are doing an awful lot of damage to the world in the name of helping it. I don't mind attacking my own fraternity because I am ashamed of it." - Kary Mullis, Inventor of the Polymerase Chain Reaction Test.

You may say, "Wait a minute, stop right there! There were more than 6 Million deaths from COVID-19. I think YOU are crazy!" - You have got to love Semmelweis! Yes, over 6 million people died between 2020 and 2022. Let us explain things according to the new medical findings of German New Medicine (GNM) and the way the PCR (Polymerase Chain Reaction) Test is used.

The PCR Test is adjustable to test positive for whatever antibody a doctor wants to detect. One could adjust the PCR test and "tune it in" to detect the antibodies of your *tears*! No wonder Dr. Kary Mullis was said to have broken down in *tears* when he heard the CDC was using the PCR test to detect and "diagnose" HIV and other fictitious viruses! The CDC and WHO are literally using the PCR test as a Weapon of Mass Destruction. That sounds unethical to us!

So why so many deaths during the pandemic? For most of us, it's hard to admit how fragile and gullible we can be, yet something combats our fragility. It's called our ego. The ego can build up a strong wall to almost anything except – *when our life is threatened.* That very threat can collapse the wall of our ego in a split second. That threat can come from a pandemic scare, a cancer diagnosis, or even the headlines in the news media! Our brain reacts like it's been hit with a "Voodoo Spell" and all we can think of is "How long do I have to live?" We could experience a "death fright scare" conflict in the terms of German New Medicine and start down the road of a disease. We are now recognizing any disease as a Significant Biological Program (SBP). And our symptoms are part of either a Conflict Active Phase or a Healing Phase, depending on what organ is having a tissue response to a mental life shock. Common sense would say: the diagnosis of testing positive for COVID-19 after taking a PCR test would scare the "breath out of anyone"! And it does. What do we do the split second we are threatened with our life? We GASP for AIR! We gasp unconsciously because our brain signals our lungs to get more oxygen to stay alive! That "Death fright scare" triggers our lungs to go into a period of cell overgrowth to "help" us cope with the life conflict. It turns into a vicious cycle if allowed to continue without resolving the emotional scare. The lungs cells overgrow and then get broken down by bacteria, then overgrow and get broken down until the lungs are too full of "diseased tissue" and fluids to stay alive. It's all been proven in German New Medicine.

From childhood, we are taught *not to question authority figures.* It would be wise to rethink that. The current medical protocols for many so-called "diseases" *hinder* a patient from *resolving* their conflicts and letting the body heal like it's designed to. The biological shock/conflict is allowed to spin on and on in the patient's psyche-brain-body. Remember, disease is not caused by germs, bacteria, or viruses. When the emotional situation is ignored, the situation slowly worsens. The doctors in hospitals are one step away from the nurses. The nurses end up dealing face-to-face with patients who have the "breath scared out of them".

In cases involving COVID-19, those very patients eventually get put on sedatives because the protocol dictates that a tube be put down their throats to be put on a respirator. If nurses don't give patients the sedative, the patient would yank out the tube! The protocols are ludicrous and delusional, yet the doctors still give the orders to nurses. What kind of insane person would knowingly do that? The hospital protocols help send these patients and their harmless souls to the grave! They have been scared to death and not allowed to resolve the threat of being diagnosed with a "you could die..." from someone they perceive as an authoritative figure which the patient views as the "Alpha Male". QUESTION EVERYTHING!

Chapter 23
What about man-made viruses?

Scientists confuse the subject with man-made viruses or biologics. The word "virus" means poison, and scientists thought that viruses (exosomes) were attacking to kill as a poison would. Frighteningly, virologists and scientists are now making man-made viruses (poisons) to kill. These are pollutants that are still not transferable by breathing or touching. Yes, they can circulate them in the atmosphere but don't be confused that they are made by your body or contagious! They are simply manipulated genetic strands that act like poison. They are not naturally occurring viruses, remember they are not alive, so they don't fly around and attack you. We mean, come on, Chinese jungle bat viruses, *really*? How do these scientists sleep at night?

Once again, if your body has any toxins present, both bacteria and viruses and often fungus may be present to *clean up* the mess and remove or repair the damaged cells. Like we wouldn't blame firemen for setting a fire at a burning house, we should not blame bacteria, viruses, or fungi for diseases. They are only trying to clean up the toxins by feeding on them to eliminate them from the diseased site or to repair and rebuild tissue that has been damaged. It's a construction site!

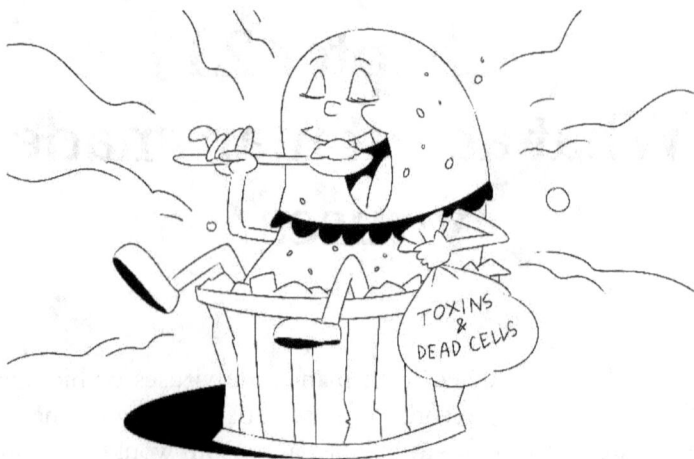

Viruses are so tiny that they can only be seen by an electron microscope and the atomic force microscope (1989). Although viruses were being blamed for diseases in the late 1800s, the electron microscope was not invented until 1931.

If scientists take a snapshot of any disease tissue and look at it under an electron microscope, they will see bits of viruses because they are like sponges, which are there for the cleanup. Scientists are witnessing dead cells with virus particles within them mixed with other dead cells (isolates) with viruses in them. They call this a virus "isolate" to make it sound as if they have something "isolated". But they don't! Again, they are presenting us with science experiments based on complete speculation and assumptions! Smoke and mirrors.

Viruses are three times smaller than an infrared ray. Their actual size is about 400 nm. This makes them 10 times smaller than a Bacterium!

Their small size makes them the perfect suspect and scapegoat for any health crime. No one could actually see them or isolate them because even an electron microscope causes what's called nano-particulates. Scientists are looking at dead cellular debris that is bigger than viruses and too difficult to distinguish with certainty, let alone isolate to test.

Doctors never see viruses because they're too small to test. So instead, they test for antibodies. *There has never, ever been a correlation between a specific virus and a specific antibody.* And antibodies will *always* be present if you have toxins in an area of the body that is being tested. It means absolutely nothing other than the body has toxins!

To this day, no one has isolated a virus. In scientific papers, a "virus isolate" is referred to. The titles of the reports sound convincing on the initial read, but when you read through the content of the report, they refer to Virus Like Particles (VLP)! That is not a virus! That is an ASSUMPTION it is a virus! And if you read further, you will note that, in many reports, this isolate has so much cellular debris added to it under a microscope it doesn't make sense! The isolate we see in the pictures includes dead tissue cells of sick animals and a hand full of other viruses. A "virus isolate" is NOT an "isolated virus". This is important because *to prove a disease, you must have an isolated virus.* Back to Koch's postulates.

What this means. And we repeat... **There has never been any virus isolated EVER!** We're going to name a few; maybe you can think of more. Measles virus, polio virus, diphtheria virus, tetanus virus, herpes virus, HIV virus. None of these have EVER been isolated.

We'll say it again:

We are on a mission. We are shifting the world into a whole new paradigm and expressing a new consciousness. By you reading this book, we can end the deception, trickery, corruption, and fraud by Big Pharma and government medical institutions who claim they are "only trying to save lives".

1954 marks the year when a scientist named John Enders essentially came up with protocols, which, when followed, would make it *appear* as if they had an "isolated virus" for any disease. Scientists can make it *appear* as if there is a new virus for any presentation within their lab.

Dr. Stefan Lanka said, **"In the course of my studies, I and others have not been able to find proof of the existence of disease-**

causing viruses anywhere." Remember, Dr. Stefan Lanka offered $100,000 to anyone who could prove that the measles virus was isolated. Dr. Stephan Lanka did a control experiment and showed that by introducing a small particle of yeast into an experiment, he could show death (Cytopathic Effect, CPE) in cell pictures that look *exactly* like the pictures from scientists *claiming* viral infection! [48]

Why is this important? Just to remind you. Because if you *can't* isolate the virus, you can't ever **prove** it causes disease. Plus, if you do any research at all, you will find that all the diseases blamed on viruses have often been diagnosed *with no* virus being present! And no control experiments are ever presented.

Facts do not cease to exist because they are ignored. -Aldous Huxley

---

In the awesome book *VIRUS MANIA*, there are over 2000 research articles saying the same thing. The book is full of facts regarding the bogus virus theory of disease. [49]

Most research is paid for by those who make money on the outcome. The French government and the church supported Louis Pasteur's research and paid him to promote germ theory and then vaccinations. And now we know his work was fraudulent!

If you look at today's research, it is paid for by Big Pharma in one way or another. There is rarely independent research, and the conclusions are bought and paid for.

Today most books on health are still written with the idea that bacteria and viruses cause disease. Unfortunately, it is an idea repeated for 150 years. Anytime you hear about a virus or a bacteria, try to think of what toxin (physical, mental, social, or spiritual) actually caused that disease process? Anytime you hear about an infection, think of what *toxin* caused the bacteria, virus or fungus to show up?

"It should be clear from this discussion that no disease is caused by a virus" - Dawn Lester and David Park, What Really Makes You Ill? [50]

"The health authorities are no longer maintaining that any virus whatsoever purportedly causing disease has been *directly proven* to exist." Dr. Robert Mendelsohn MD [51]

"Life is an incredibly complex interdependence of matter and energy among millions of species beyond and within our own skin." - Dr. Margulis [52]

"This germ theory of the Dark Age is nothing, but a deliberate *mass insanity* pushed upon society to gain profit and power. By acting against microbes as a medical establishment dictate, one is actually helping to dig one's own grave, while paying someone else to show where to dig. This insanity must end." - Dr. William Trebing [53]

We realize this all sounds incredible! When we were doing research, we were amazed this was all factually proven. Not once has a virus ever been isolated as the cause of these diseases. Whenever scientists talk about isolating a virus, there are always a bunch of fancy words to cover up the fact that they didn't isolate the virus. Word salad once again!

Even the American Center of Disease Control (CDC) admitted they never isolated the coronavirus. Even the dreaded HIV virus was never isolated! Nor was polio or the measles virus or any other virus for that matter. Yes, you can see viruses, but they have NEVER been isolated. Viruses are the perfect scapegoat for any disease because they are commonly *present to help the cells survive.*

We were all led to believe in school that these "bad germs" are single-minded opportunists that work for your persistent demise. Nothing could be further from the truth. They are part of the body's defense mechanism to clean house and purify the system and return us to homeostasis (balance). They exist in their granular form until needed.

Chapter 24
What about kids getting Polio?

There have been several attempts scientifically to prove that you *can* catch a virus. **The only thing that research shows is that you can't catch anything!**

We will admit this next part might be sensitive to some readers.

Scientists tried to prove that polio is contagious by doing extensive studies on monkeys. *They finally resorted to <u>drilling a hole</u> in a monkey's skull and injecting a ground-up piece of spinal cord from a sick child with polio into the monkey's brain.* When the monkey became paralyzed, they reported that they succeeded in showing polio was contagious! You would think it highly rare that any of us have to worry about having an open hole in our skull. Drilling a hole in someone's head would paralyze anyone! Therefore, it's safe to say, polio is NOT contagious.

A cornerstone for the polio virus theory was started in 1908 by scientists Karl Landsteiner and Erwin Popper. The WHO claimed their experiments were a milestone in the obliteration of polio. Listen to the account of the ridiculous experiments used to validate the use of polio vaccines!

> Landsteiner and Popper took a diseased piece of spinal marrow from a lame nine-year-old boy. They chopped it up, dissolved it in water, and injected one or two whole cups of it into the *abdominal cavities* of two test monkeys: one died and the other became permanently paralyzed. (97), (98) Their studies were plagued by a

mind-boggling range of basic problems. First, the "glop" they poured into the animals was not even infectious since the paralysis didn't appear in the monkeys and guinea pigs given the alleged "virus soup" to *drink* or in those that had it *injected* into their extremities. (99) [54]

Shortly after, researchers Simon Flexner and Paul Lewis experimented with a comparable mixture, **injecting this into monkeys' brains. (100)** [55] **Next, they brewed a new soup from the brains of these monkeys and put the mix into another monkey's head. This monkey indeed became ill!**

But this experiment shows no proof of a viral infection! The glop used cannot be termed an isolated virus, even with all the will in the world!! Nobody could have seen any virus, as the electron microscope wasn't invented until 1931! Also, Flexner and Lewis did not disclose the ingredients of their "injection soup." By 1948, it was still unknown "how the polio virus invades humans," as expert John Paul of Yale University stated at an international poliomyelitis congress in New York City (102) [56]

Believe it or not, this is the ONE experiment that is held up as *proving* that polio is caused by a virus that invades humans! They injected the goop soup into a monkey's brain to cause paralysis and thus link polio to a virus!

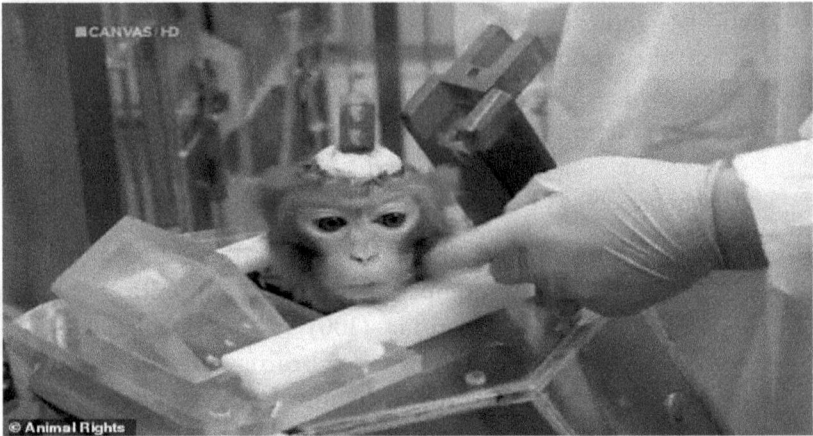

However, not all scientists were impressed.

In 1941, expert scientists reported in the scientific journal ARCHIVES of Pediatrics that "Human poliomyelitis **has not** been shown conclusively to be a *contagious disease*." [57] Well, if anyone read the previous experiment, they should ALL conclude that!

In 1955, Salk's Vaccine was celebrated nationwide as a substance that protected against polio outbreaks. However, in 1954, Bernice Eddy, who oversaw the US government 's vaccine safety tests, reported that the Salk vaccine *had caused severe paralyses in test monkeys*. How do they solve that finding? Eddy was shortly after made to *give up* her polio research.

Within only two weeks, the number of polio cases among vaccinated children had climbed to nearly 200. In May 1955, Carl Eklund, the US government's highest authority on viruses, said, "only vaccinated children had been afflicted by polio. And only in areas where no polio cases had been reported for close to a year! In nine out of ten cases, paralysis for the polio vaccine appeared in the injected arm. In New York, Rhode Island, and Wisconsin, the number of cases of paralysis jumped to 500% after vaccine programs were administered. Most frequently in the arm which was given the shot!" [58]

Guess what Polio, Aseptic Meningitis, the Flu, Lyme Disease, Pneumonia, Lupus, and AIDS (Acquired Immune Deficiency

Syndrome) all have in common? The answer is: *THEY ALL HAVE IDENTICAL SYMPTOMS*!! The only difference between them is that their symptoms are *switched around* a bit in the order of what symptom is listed first when referenced in any popular diagnostic text. Essentially, all these diseases are part of the same process, which renders them practically identical.

Chapter 25
So, what did cause Polio?

The truth about Polio is that the government sprayed yards, orchards, and parks with a DDT pesticide (glyphosates) that killed moths from the late 1940s to early 1950s. This was a *lead-arsenate* toxic concoction that is known to cause nerve and muscle damage exactly like the "Polio" symptoms. Lucky for us, they stopped spraying *yards* with this toxic chemical in 1955. And lucky *and profitable* for Big Pharma, they came up with a Polio vaccine right at the end of the time they stopped spraying (1955) so they could claim that the Polio vaccine was a success.

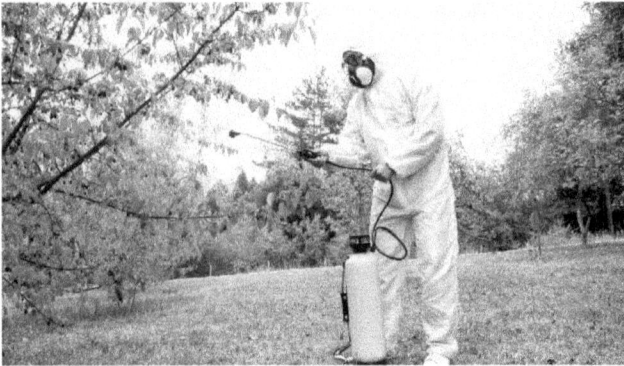

The other thing they cleverly did was force doctors to change their diagnostic tactics. Any child after 1959 with polio-like symptoms was to be diagnosed with AFP (Acute Flaccid Paralysis). "Doctors are instructed not to look for the polio virus itself, as 'the virus is very hard to find.' Instead, this task is to be left to WHO and the other governmental agencies that inspect turds (doctors are to send in two). This would've been comical if it were not so tragically deceptive," says Janine Roberts in *Fear of the Invisible: A Hidden Epidemic.* [59]

She continues with, "Under these new rules, patients previously diagnosed with paralytic polio were re-diagnosed. When patients in Detroit, diagnosed as having paralytic polio during 1958 epidemic, were re-tested as required by the new rule, 49% were found not to have polio virus and were therefore told they did not have polio. I did not know how to characterize this except as an incredible act of medical fraud." [60] So much for polio vaccines eradicating polio. They only eradicated the diagnosis and continued the shell game!

"Health officials convinced the Chinese to rename the bulk of their polio to Guillain-Barré Syndrome (GBS). A study found that the new disorder (Chinese Paralytic syndrome) and GBS was really polio. After mass vaccination in 1971, reports of polio went down but GBS increased about 10-fold! In the WHO polio vaccine eradication in the Americas, there were 930 cases of paralytic disease all called polio. Five years later, at the end of the campaign, *roughly 2000 cases of paralytic disease occurred but only 6 of them were called polio.* The rate of paralytic disease doubled, but the disease definition changed so drastically that hardly any of it was called polio anymore." *Vaccination*, Greg Beattie. [61]

Unfortunately, government agencies and corporations continue to spray these nerve poisons all over the world as herbicides and pesticides and cause neurological problems in children. [62]

The inventor of the polio vaccine Jonas Salk is quoted as saying that over two-thirds of the polio cases after 1976 were caused by his Salk vaccine! [63]

Chapter 26
What about the Spanish Flu of 1918 that killed 20-50 million?

This next bit of information will REALLY knock your socks off!

There was a study by the Boston Public health department in 1918 *to* prove that the Spanish flu was contagious. We have all heard that the Spanish flu killed 20,000,000 to 50,000,000 people. The study was done on 100 healthy, "volunteer" Navy sailors doing time for some infraction. Three tests were performed.

One contagion test had the volunteers exposed face to face within inches of a sick person with Spanish flu. At the end of ten minutes, they were to inhale while the sick individual blew as hard as they could into the sailor's mouth. Another test was done by swabbing the volunteer sailors in the eyes, nose and mouth with the mucus concoction from those infected. And yet another test was done by injecting them with the goop of those that were sick with Spanish Flu.

NOT ONE SAILOR CAME DOWN WITH THE SPANISH FLU! - Invisible Rainbow by Arthur Firstenberg. [64] How do you explain that?

The Spanish flu was NOT contagious. Yes, many people died but it was not caused by a contagious virus (because viruses or bacteria are NOT contagious, nor do they cause disease)! There were so many culprits other than a virus. The most likely being the extreme stress caused by the announcement of WWI combined with a bacterial meningitis vaccine containing mercury, aluminum, and other toxins. This vaccine was given to millions both in our country and around the world. The radio wave was first released around the world in 1917 with the invention of new radar equipment. There were extreme sanitation problems and little nutrition due to the abysmal food supply following the war.

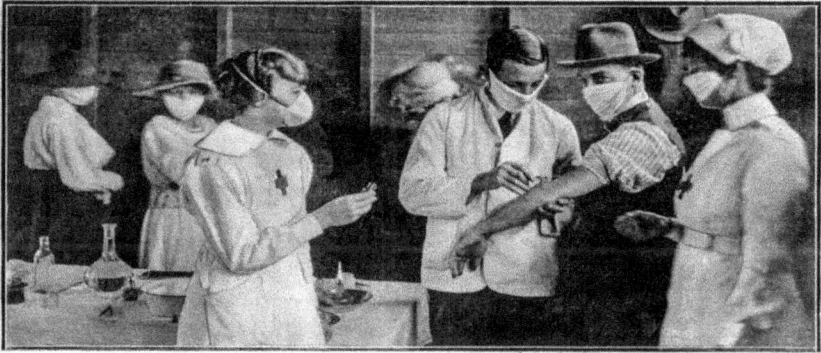

And guess what? The Spanish flu did not start in Spain. They were the only country uncensored during WWI, so they were the only country reporting deaths. And one reason the Spanish Flu has never been corrected is that it helps disguise the origin of the pandemic.

This next revelation could be a shock to hear...

We know the origin of the pandemic involved a **vaccine experiment** on US soldiers, the US much prefers to label it The Spanish Flu instead of The Fort Riley Vaccine of 1918, or something similar. The Spanish Flu possibly started at Fort Riley, Kansas, where this experimental vaccine was given by the Rockefeller Institute. The Rockefeller Institute was established back in 1901.

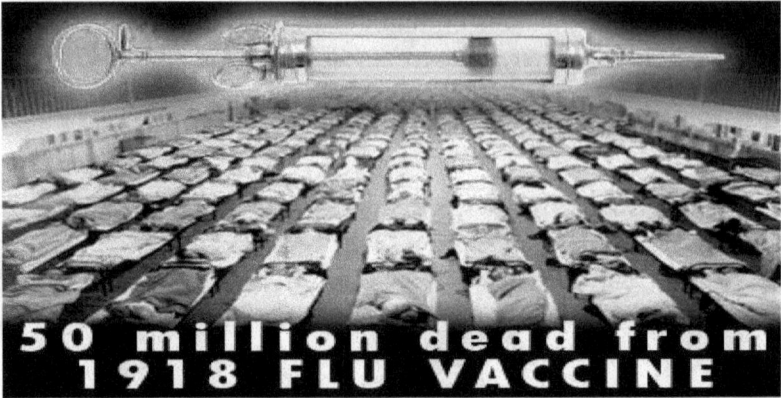

50 million dead from 1918 FLU VACCINE

"The American Rockefeller Institute for Medical Research and its experimental bacterial meningococcal vaccine may have killed 50-100 million people in 1918-19" is a far less effective sales slogan than the overly simplistic 'vaccines save lives'." – Kevin Barry, the President of First Freedoms, Inc. a 501.c.3. He is a former federal attorney, a representative at the United Nations Headquarters in New York, and the author of "Vaccine Whistleblower: Exposing Autism Research Fraud at the CDC". [65]

Check out www.firstfreedoms.org

Remember that bacteria and viruses will appear whenever toxins are present? If you were unfortunate enough to be a soldier or part of the military staff in 1918, you would have been injected with the experimental bacterial meningitis vaccine. The experimental vaccine, derived from horses, comprised toxins like mercury and aluminum, along with horse serum. When you're injected with toxins, you're bound to feel sick. Combining the heavy metals in the vaccines with the newly released worldwide radio wave of electricity was deadly.

And that was reported again and again. Nausea, diarrhea, vomiting, and often death... makes sense, right? So, did the vaccinations stop? No, of course not, the Rockefeller Institute for Health kindly sent vaccinations overseas to "help" the rest of the world. And why not when you have no care for anyone? If it was profitable and deadly in the US, it was bound to have the same results in other countries. You might think they didn't mind killing people!

There were far more deaths from the Spanish flu than from any actual war. If there was any desire to reduce the world population and make money, vaccines were successful. The Rockefeller Institute of "Health" had discovered vaccines were better for business than war. They could *appear as if they were helping people* yet be killing them. Remember, if you reverse Live, it spells Evil.

Another major culprit was the HUGE amount of fear and emotional trauma that can affect large numbers of people simultaneously and make them sick.

Have you noticed there has never been another Spanish flu viral epidemic? Because it was a made-up flu virus! You will have to look for the references in the back to research this on your own. Google has removed a lot of information about the Spanish flu after the coronavirus was *announced*, but it may still be uncensored at www.duckduckgo.com

If you have gotten vaccines in your life, we are happy you have not had any complications. However, there is a multitude of evidence that vaccines have caused many deaths. It's muted and hidden from the public. Most people have never heard of VAERS (Vaccine Adverse Events Reporting System). It is the government website to report adverse reactions after getting a vaccine. The first glaring issue with the concept of having a reporting system is that it is voluntary!

Chapter 27
What about the HIV and AIDS epidemic?

Guess what? There are over 1500 peer-reviewed articles *disputing* the assertion that an HIV virus is linked to AIDS (Acquired Immune Deficiency Syndrome) or that there *ever was* an HIV virus in the first place! Look at www.virusmyth.org and www.virusmyth.com for more research. According to the book *Virus Mania*, there are so many researchers, including the "discoverers" of the HIV virus (theory), Luc Montagnier and Robert Gallo, who have admitted that there *never* was an HIV retrovirus or virus that could be identified! [66]

"Up to today there is no single scientifically convincing evidence for the existence of HIV. Not even one such a retrovirus has been isolated and purified by the methods of classical virology." Dr. Heinz Ludwig Sanger, Emeritus Professor of Molecular Biology and Virology, Max-Planck-Institute for Biochemistry, Munich. [67]

Listen to this deception! In May 1983, doctors of the Institute Pasteur in France reported that they had isolated a new virus, which they suggested might cause AIDS... But, seven years later, "Dr. Ulrich Marcus, the press spokesman of the Robert Koch Institute reported that the HIV-virus cannot be isolated" District Court of Dortmund, Germany- Stefan Lanka and K. Krafeld, taken from the book, *Vaccination. Genocide in the Third Millennium?* [68]

In 1984, Robert Gallo published four articles in Science along with others, *claiming* he had isolated the HIV virus and concluding that it was the probable cause of AIDS. Several years later, *Robert Gallo*, HIV virus "discoverer," along with thirty-seven legal, medical and research professionals sent a letter to the journal, *Science*, asking it to *officially retract* the original four papers making the case for HIV as the cause of AIDS. According to the letter's authors *widespread evidence has now emerged that the studies were not only poorly carried out, but that their results* **were falsified***!!*

Along with a copy of the handwritten changes, the letter from the thirty-seven experts *includes* a letter from Robert Gallo himself, *admitting that HIV could not be isolated from human samples* alone, and a letter from an electron microscope expert saying that there was **no HIV virus contained in Gallo's 1984 samples."**

Dr. Kary Mullis, Nobel Prize winner for the PCR test in 1993, states, *"If there is proof that HIV is the cause of AIDS, there should be scientific documents which either singly or collectively demonstrate that fact, at least with a high probability. There is no such document."* [69]

In 1996, *Luc Montagnier*, one of the other "discoverers" of the HIV virus admitted in the documentary *AIDS-The Doubt*, *"There is no scientific proof that HIV causes AIDS."*

Reinharth Kurth, director of the Robert Koch Institute, which as the leader in AIDS research, conceded in Der Speigel, (September 9th, 2004), *"We don't exactly know how HIV causes disease."* [70]

Walter Gilbert, Nobel Prize winner in microbiology at Harvard University, stated in 1989 that "he would not be surprised if there were another cause of AIDS and even that HIV was not involved." He also stated, "The major thing that concerns me by calling HIV the cause of AIDS IS THAT WE DO NOT HAVE PROOF OF CAUSATION." [71]

The largest and best-conceived study about sex and AIDS shows that AIDS is not a sexually transmitted disease! Nancy Padian's 1997 "Study on Seroconversion Rates Among Couples", in the Journal of American Medical Association states, "the fact is glaringly obvious in the most comprehensive paper on this topic in it **not a single case could be uncovered in which an HIV negative partner eventually became positive through sexual contact with his or her or HIV positive partner."** That is to say, the observed transmission rate was zero.

Dr. Root-Bernstein is a physiologist at Michigan State University and the author of the book *Rethinking AIDS*. "When I look at AIDS patients, I can find that no one who develops AIDS that does not have a multitude of immunosuppressant agents working on them simultaneously. The logic of the war on AIDS is seriously flawed." [72]

When he was asked what would happen if an otherwise healthy person was exposed to the HIV virus, he said, "There are people who are married to blood transfusion patients, people who are married to hemophiliacs, who have been exposed to HIV from these means. There are surgeons who cut themselves all the time while working on AIDS patients, and all these people are free of HIV." Nothing would happen. [73]

A 1993 national TV special on mainstream television did a special feature, "What is the Real Cause of AIDS. The show began by stating that HIV and AIDS have no proven correlation. It then switched to *"the man with the deep pockets in the AIDS establishment,"* Dr. Anthony Fauci. Dr. Fauci, then director of the National Institute of Allergy and Infectious Disease, said, "What's next is to develop an appropriate, safe and effective therapy, and a safe and effective vaccine. That's the bottom line of it. You have a disease, you identify the cause, you identify a treatment, and you get a vaccine for it". [74] Again, the ONLY OPTION he presented was to push a VACCINE! Ulterior motive, anyone??

Hmmm, do you hear anything familiar to the trillion-dollar COVID -19 vaccine agenda?

The AIDS symptoms in our country more likely stemmed from either fear or subsequent testing and treatments (see www.learninggnm.com.). [75] Or from "new" recreational drugs (like poppers or inhalants). These were "new" drugs with strong side effects used by many homosexuals.

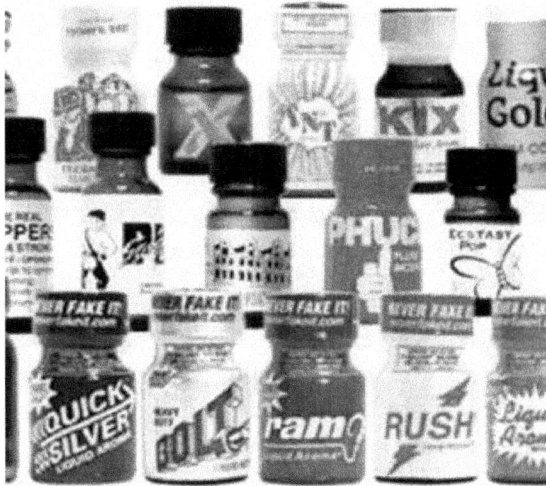

Poppers became very popular in the late 1970s. Sales added up to $50,000,000 in 1976 in just one state! "By 1977, poppers had permeated every angle of gay life, and in 1979, more than 5,000,000 people consumed poppers more than once a week." writes Harry Haverkos, who joined the CDC in 1981 and was the leading official during the AIDS movement.

Poppers have side effects known to severely damage the immune system, genes, lungs, liver, heart and brain; they can produce neural damage similar to that of multiple sclerosis, or can have carcinogenic effects, and can lead to "sudden sniffing death." And the medical industry knew about its various dangers.

In 1981, the New England Journal of Medicine published several articles at the same time pointing out the use of drugs and the fast-lane lifestyle as a possible cause of AIDS. Besides the widespread use of poppers and nitrate inhalants, this lifestyle often included many other toxic drugs. Hang in there with this list or jump to the next paragraph. (You won't hurt our feelings!) Those drugs include crystal meth, cocaine, crack, barbiturates, ecstasy, heroin, Librium, LSD Mandrex, MDA, MDM, mescaline, mushrooms, purple haze, Seconal, special K, Tuinal, THC, PCP, STP, DMT, SDK, WDW, window pane, blotter, orange, sunshine, sweet pea, sky blue, Christmas tree dust, Benzedrine, Dexedrine,

Dexamyl, Desoxyn, Clogidal, Nesperan, Tytch, nestex, black beauty, certyn, preludin with B12, zayl, quaalude, Nembutal, amytal, phenobarbital, Elavil, valium, darvon, mandrax, opium, stidyl, halidax, caldfyn, optimal and drayl. [76]

The fast lane of the homosexual lifestyle often included a poor diet and long-term use of antibiotics and anti-fungal substances, which damage the mitochondria (and mitochondria are the bacterial powerhouses of the cells)!

The HIV scare started with five seriously ill gay men in 1981. Gottleib, a scientist from the University of California, brought these five men together after searching for several months to create a link. The men had had no contact with each other; however, it was speculated that they had gotten ill from sexual contact (go figure, small details to overlook they had never met).

The CDC found this "discovery" an *opportunity to create a whole new epidemic* since research funding for proving viruses caused cancer was soon running out. There was a widespread media message that caused the belief and panic that a deadly contagious sexually transmitted epidemic occurring, at least among gay men. "Even though there was no scientific data to back these perceptions up. The CDC, the gay community, as well as the pharmaceutical companies were also behind suppressing any information that drugs were causing AIDS.

Guess what? The CDC set on the search for a deadly virus and even tried to hide data. In 1982, the CDC's own AIDS expert, Harry Haverkos analyzed three drugs, including poppers and concluded that the drugs did play a weighty role in AIDS. But the CDC refused to publish their own high-ranking employee's study. Haverkos transferred to the FDA in 1984 to become an AIDS coordinator there. In 1985 the paper finally appeared in the journal *Sexually Transmitted Diseases*, Haverkos, Harry, Disease Manifestation among Homosexual Men with Acquired Immunodeficiency Syndrome: A Possible Role of Nitrites in Kaposi's Sarcoma, *Sexually Transmitted Diseases*, October- December 1985, pp. 203-208. [77]

The Wall Street Journal published an article stating that ***drug abuse was so common among AIDS patients that this, and not the HIV virus, must be considered the primary cause of AIDS*** [78]

In Africa, AIDS became a catch-all diagnosis for any number of symptoms common to many other diseases. Or better yet, there were many diseases linked under the term AIDS. There was no universal definition of AIDS (Acquired Immune Deficiency Syndrome). So, anyone suffering from many non-specific symptoms like weight loss, diarrhea and itching was labeled an AIDS diagnosis. The HIV/AIDS epidemic is actually a smorgasbord of well-known diseases, many of which correlate closely with poverty. [79]

Chapter 28
What about all the positive HIV tests?

The HIV antibody testing used has some huge issues with false positives. Nobel Prize winner Kary Mullis, known for inventing the PCR test used for COVID-19, states, *"They got some big numbers for HIV-positive people in Africa before they realized that antibodies to malaria -which everyone in Africa has- shows up as HIV positive on tests."* [80] And not only malaria but also dozens of other typical illnesses like chronic fever, weight loss, diarrhea, and tuberculosis *all* cause HIV positive test results.

T-Cells are "immune system" cells produced by the Thymus. T-Cells can vary from day to day. One way doctors were flagrantly passing out AIDS diagnoses was to label anyone in Africa with a low T-Cell count as an AIDS patient! Isn't that ludicrous?!?

Max Essex, who is said to be one of the founding fathers of AIDS science, observed that lepers reacted positively to the HIV test. He pointed out that the results of the tests should be taken with a grain of salt.

The tragic consequences of an HIV-positive AIDS diagnosis meant that often African villagers were banished from their village to struggle with their illness alone. This often meant starvation and death.

Nevell Hodgkinson, a medical correspondent for the *Sunday Times,* spent weeks traveling through Africa. He says, "When I asked people what disease they were dying of, they replied: 'from AIDS,' whereupon I inquired: 'But from which disease in particular?' To this, they said: "This patient has tuberculosis, that one chronic diarrhea, this one malaria and that one leprosy', all diseases that have been known in Africa for ages. But then everything was re-diagnosed as AIDS out of fear of AIDS." [81]

Dr. Peter Duesberg is a pioneering virologist at the University of California at Berkley. He said, "I would drink HIV-infested water all day long. There would be absolutely no risk in doing so. **There is no proof that HIV causes AIDS.** In addition, I am familiar with retroviruses, how they begin and what they do, and on those counts, I am confident enough that HIV, no matter how, couldn't cause AIDS." He says many researchers *know that truth* but can't afford to speak up. He states, "Many people tell me that they can't afford to speak up now because their research plans and grant money depend on HIV. (They say) If I join you, my grants will be terminated just like yours." [82]

Chapter 29
What caused all the *deaths* from AIDS?

The AZT (chemotherapy) treatments and other drugs used for AIDS as well as the emotional shock and stress of the AIDS diagnosis given with a positive HIV test were the cause of the majority of deaths.

Dr. Anthony Fauci, the most powerful AIDS official, refused to be interviewed regarding the lack of evidence that AZT had *any* positive outcome. Dr. Fauci has a long history of deception. *AZT was a known chemotherapy-like medication extremely deadly to all the recipients in the one study done to validate it called the "Fischl study"!*

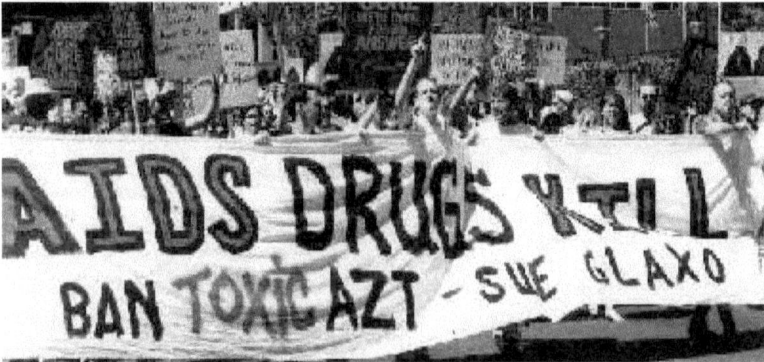

Basketball player Earvin "Magic" Johnson was one of the most famous survivors of the AZT prescription. He admits he took AZT for only a short time due to its horrible side effects. Thankfully, he never followed his doctor's advice, and he regained his health despite his HIV-positive diagnosis. He has been quoted as saying, "There is no magic in AZT, and there is no AZT in Magic." [83]

Unfortunately, The Russian Rudolph Nureyev, held by many to be the greatest ballet dancer of all time, also took AZT at the end of the 1980s. Nureyev was HIV positive, but otherwise, he was healthy. His personal physician, Dr. Michel Canesi warned him about the deadly effects of AZT, but Nureyev was too scared to stop the drug. He died in 1993.

Sadly, famed tennis star Author Ashe followed his doctors' wishes. He never stopped his treatment despite saying that "standard treatments such as AZT actually make matters worse." He died at age 36.

Dr. Stefan Lanka, expert virologist, states, "No particle of HIV has ever been obtained pure, free of contaminants nor has a complete piece of HIV RNA (or the transcribed DNA) ever been proved to exist." [84]

Over 20 million people have died of an "AIDS" diagnosis and/or treatments. Many would contend that AIDS symptoms represent any number of toxins or illnesses that were present before the *invention* of AIDS. Patients were labeled as having AIDS when, in all reality, it could have been anything that caused a toxic reaction since every single symptom of AIDS is also that of toxicity.

The United Nations predicted that ninety million Africans would die of AIDS by 2025. It looks like they haven't been as successful as they had planned.

On January 13, 2016, WHO actually *admitted* that the smallpox vaccine created AIDS/HIV in Africa.

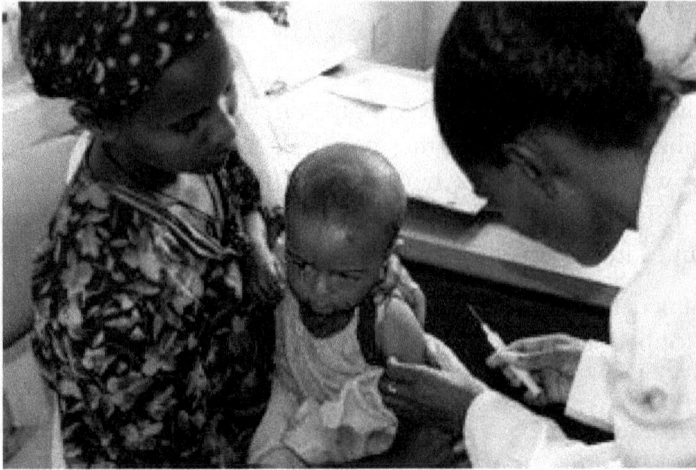

The hepatitis B vaccine was also used by millions in African countries. This vaccine was full of toxins. When the populations exhibited AIDS symptoms after reacting to the toxins in the vaccine, they were given AZT. And death followed soon after the treatment. Remember, AZT is a chemotherapeutic agent with extreme toxicity! INSANITY YET AGAIN!!

Dr. Ryke Hamer, MD, states, "AIDS is a combination of symptoms that existed already long before the invention of AIDS."

Chapter 30
What's the truth about the coronavirus?

As in today's pandemic, there is no scientific proof that COVID-19 is contagious or that it is caused by a virus! There simply isn't proof because Big Pharma stands to lose A LOT OF money if people knew the truth and were not afraid! There are many poison-like genetically engineered vaccines now made to increase the wealth of all those involved with the coronavirus since it was invented.

"If you want to predict the future, invent it." - Big Pharma

On December 16, 2019, Moderna brought their finished coronavirus vaccine to the University of North Carolina. What? Didn't we hear about something from China officially in January 2020? You might wonder what kind of crystal ball helped Moderna out. It seems as if all the countries were getting ready for a big pandemic. War games and dress rehearsals!

In 2018 there were millions of dollars spent on COVID-19 Diagnostic Test instruments and apparatus kits. The EU, Denmark, United States, Uruguay, Germany, Japan, Singapore all had large purchases two years before the official "outbreak". [85]

The Chinese Wuhan lab is owned by GlaxoSmithKline (GSK). GlaxoSmithKline owns 68% of Pfizer. Pfizer manages financials for Black Rock and made a trillion-dollar COVID-19 vaccine for us!

We found another suspicious "fact checker" on the internet. It is interesting that Reuters, a multi-million dollar and multi-national media conglomerate, has a partnership with Black Rock. Black Rock owns 8%

of Pfizer and 6.8% of AstraZeneca. Reuters, which controls a lot of the media, has a fact checker in its editorial department that oversees *removing all things negative* regarding vaccines and COVID-19 on all social media.

Let's talk about fact-checkers. These people simply don't know the basics of science. The very basics of disease-causing research are completely ignored, and for a good reason. They don't want any science that doesn't fit their narrative. Remember Koch's four postulates and the expanded version in River's six postulates?

Let's cut right to River's expanded version of six postulates from 1937.

River's Postulates are:

1. The virus can be isolated from a diseased organism

2. The virus can be cultivated and made to grow cells of a new organism

3. Proof of filterability—the virus can be separated from a medium that also contains bacteria

4. The filtered virus will produce a comparable disease when the cultivated virus is used to infect experimental animals.

5. The virus can be re-isolated from the infected experimental animal.

6. A specific immune response to the virus can be detected. [86]

Although Rivers' postulates were expanded, to this day, NO DISEASE HAS EVER BEEN PROVEN WITH THEM! Even though these are the "gold standard", and they make sense to all scientists, we'll repeat NO DISEASE HAS EVER BEEN PROVEN WITH THEM (including coronavirus)!!

The steps that scientists have taken to isolate a coronavirus are as follows. We'll let **YOU** determine how isolated this can be. [87]

1. Take a spit sample from a sick patient with a cough.

2. Centrifuge and take the cellular part (which supposedly has the virus) and leave the liquid.

3. This is called "purification"!! This goop of centrifuged cells.

4. Take this "purification" of God-only-knows-what and add it to monkey kidney cells.

5. Grow this concoction until there is enough cellular material to work with.

6. Centrifuge again and examine under an electron microscope.

Seriously? This is the virus isolation method used?? If you read this, you can see how there is NO WAY they would know if what they are looking at came from the cells of the animal or the cells of the patient! Plus, they don't have a purified or isolated virus in any sense of the word!

Another research study that researchers have used as proof that a *coronavirus causes a disease* is:

1. Take the nose mucus of sick people

2. Grow this snot with a mixture of monkey kidney cells.

3. Centrifuge this crazy mixture

4. Inject this "purification" of cellular mix into two monkeys.

One monkey developed pneumonia, and the other had some sort of respiratory symptoms related to respiratory disease. And that, my friend, is so-called proof that a "coronavirus" can cause disease! Can you see how anything in the mixture could cause the disease?

No study has proven that coronavirus, or *any virus* is disease-causing or contagious, nor has any study proven anything except that virologists are a misguided group of people!

Why do they have so many pictures? Because they have *talented graphics artists* and *computer-generated images* that make wonderful artwork. An electron microscope can't be used to look at anything living, and the images are *always grainy black and white*. Thus, there is no evidence that the virus is entering the cell or "infecting" it, and the color images are all graphics. The live images from the atomic force microscope research prove that the viruses (exosomes) are *leaving* the cell to help it.

As far as contagion studies, there are not any that prove contagion but rather the OPPOSITE! You can look at your own experience. We all know someone who said they had the COVID virus or tested positive (with some antibody test), and their spouse or family members had no issues. Rarely does any of us even know of anyone who died unless they were old or sick. We all know someone who felt VERY toxic with something they called COVID-19. So, yes, there were toxins designed to make us sick. But they are man-made *by design*.

When the labs are "making a virus," the only thing they can do is put together genetic coding strands to produce a protein. They cannot genetically change a virus since they can't even isolate one! Another important thing to remember as you frantically clean your hands and surfaces to "kill" a virus is that *viruses aren't living*! They are non-living nano particulates that are mRNA or part DNA strands surrounded by a protein, and THEY ARE NOT ALIVE. That means viruses don't move, they don't replicate, and they don't fly. They inject themselves into a cell to "infect" it. But guess what? They are already there.

Spider-Man is not real. He is not coming to put an end to the deception. But YOU can start BELIEVING that germs, bacteria, fungi, and viruses are NOT AT WAR IN OUR BODIES. We can all stop believing in the Germ Theory and stop believing viruses are deadly!

As the inventor of the PCR test, Kary Mullis, tells us again and again, even back with HIV,

"A PCR test should *never* be a tool in the *diagnosis of infectious diseases*." [88] Every package on a PCR Test has this statement printed on it! And recall, the PCR tests are adjustable! As we mentioned, Kary Mullis died in August 2019 before he could discredit Dr. Fauci and the WHO for using the PCR tests extensively to diagnose coronavirus. You should know, Mullis was adamantly against all things Dr. Fauci due to the HIV fraud.

Remember hearing about the president of Tanzania, Africa, named John Magufuli, that said fruit and goats tested positive for COVID-19 when sent secretly to a lab? Apparently, he realized something the rest of the world did not about the testing. Magufuli died of a cardiac arrest shortly after making those revelations. Does his death sound suspicious?

The WHO, CDC, NIH, and Dr. Fauci are all under investigation for their part in creating a huge epidemic scare with no scientific proof. The total mortality rate and risk come up at less than a normal flu year. Oh, we're sure Big Pharma thought they would be more successful at creating their deadly COVID-19 toxins. They have produced some very dangerous vaccine gene therapy and a scared and compliant population.

Also, it is intriguing that there are coronavirus *patents* before 2019. You can research on the non-censored DuckDuckGo.com search platform. We all know if you want to patent something, you can *as long as it doesn't come from Mother Nature.*

Bottom line, you cannot breathe on someone and kill them, and neither will junior or grandma. That is a man-made fairy tale that has no basis in the scientific method!

We realize this may be disturbing. You may want to dismiss everything we're saying up to this point and after as pure conspiracy theory. However, it may be easier to *believe* for your own peace of mind, that Mother Nature, God, Divine, whatever label you want, has a higher plan than to make her/his children *scared to death of a deadly virus.* And the higher plan is to reveal the truth with your common sense and intuition! Bacteria, fungi, AND viruses are **HELPFUL**.

Yes, you or your friend may have come down with some flu-like symptoms very horrible. That simply means you were "highly toxic" with something your body really didn't like and needed to purge. The COVID-19 pandemic, according to the stats, is about as deadly as the normal flu.

"COVID-19 is not the problem; it is a problem, one largely solvable with early treatments that are safe, effective, and inexpensive. The problem is endemic corruption in the medical industrial complex, currently supported at every turn by mass media companies. This cartel's coup d'état has already siphoned billions from taxpayers, already vacuumed up trillions from the global middle class, and created the excuse for massive propaganda, censorship, and control worldwide. Along with its captured regulators, this cartel has ushered in the global war on freedom and democracy." - Robert F. Kennedy Jr. from "The Real Anthony Fauci" [89]

Chapter 31
What's the word on COVID-19 contagion? Can you actually catch a germ?

The only thing contagious is the emotional shock that families or nations may face together as in stress or tension or fear or arguments. Or they also may face the same toxicity in their environment in man-made biological weapons, electrical EMFs, man-made food, or as air pollution (like glyphosate insecticides and chemtrails).

You can be sleeping near your spouse, children, or relatives who are sick, and often you don't get sick. You've heard of someone who's tested positive for coronavirus, and they made no one else sick even though they were quarantined together. Yes, people in the same family or at the same job sometimes get sick at the same time. And that's because they are experiencing the same toxins or life conflicts at the same time. So, the body's response is *to get flu-like symptoms or cold symptoms to get rid of the toxins* through the lungs, urine, poop or skin. How amazing is your body! It's always working to keep you healthy!! Even when we toxify it repeatedly.

So, if there are no studies showing that you can catch anything, either bacterial or viral or fungal, why don't they do some more? Because you can't catch anything! RESEARCH WILL RARELY FUND ANY STUDY UNLESS IT'S GOING TO MAKE SOMEONE A **PROFIT**.

No virus or bacteria is contagious from another person. Not breathing on you. Not hugging. Not kissing. Not coughing. Not even having sex! These diseases you're thinking up all have a scientific explanation that starts with a toxin, either spiritual, mental, emotional, physical or chemical!!

That doesn't mean there isn't something in the air like 5G, or in the environment, or on the surfaces, or in the water, or in the food, or in stress... there are toxins everywhere. But toxins and germs are different. MAN-MADE VIRUSES ARE ALSO TOXINS!

Toxins don't fly around and TRY to kill you or make you sick. Toxins cannot be avoided, and toxic events cannot be avoided. But they can be identified and dealt with before they turn into a disease. This is why there are many things on the planet that nature provides for us to remove the toxins from our bodies. And one of the best ways to stay healthy is to recognize when something toxic has occurred to our psyche or our physical body. **Cleansing toxins spiritually (i.e., forgiveness), mentally (i.e., letting go of bad memories), emotionally (i.e., releasing anger) and physically (i.e., fasting) is a key to being healthy!**

Chapter 32
What about the testing?

PCR tests, Antibody tests, and every other test for a coronavirus are surrogate tests. This means they have NEVER been compared to any "gold standard". This means they are completely useless. If you don't have a definitive negative or positive to compare a test to, then all results of positive or negative are USELESS.

We don't want to spend any time on this other than to give you another quote from the *inventor* of the PCR test, which says it all. Kary Mullis, the inventor of the PCR test, has insisted time and time again, *"You cannot use the PCR test to prove causation from a virus and it cannot be used to diagnose illness."*

Ask yourself if it seems very odd that Kary Mullis, PCR test inventor, died of strange causes right before the start of the COVID-19 pandemic!

A file from March 30, 2020, from the CDC and the FDA concedes: "Detection of viral RNA may not indicate the presence of an infectious virus or that 2019-nCoV is the causative agent for clinical symptoms" and "This test cannot rule out diseases caused by other bacterial or viral pathogens." So why has this test been used extensively to determine how many deaths and cases there are from the pandemic? Because they want to INSTILL FEAR TO SELL THE VACCINES! They create and plan out their agenda with so many tax dollars the agenda becomes TOO BIG TO FAIL in their minds! Gates, Fauci, and Big Pharma companies stockpile their vaccines by the billions. Their agenda is to sell their supply and make a profit. They understand "units" (to sell). That is why they have to *instill fear in everyone*. It's like cattle herding; once cattle are scared enough, they can be directed to where the rancher wants them to go. Are you shouting "conspiracy theorists" at us, or is it a Semmelweis Reflex you're having? Let's end the mass deception.

FDA quote, "positive results do not rule out bacterial infection or co-infection with other viruses. The agent detected may not be the definite cause of disease."

Light Mix Modular SARS-CoV Assays are another test used. Here's their announcement, "These *assays are NOT intended for use as an aid in the diagnosis or coronavirus infection.*"

Seriously? Using those tests makes as much sense as being required to wear "protective" masks that come from a box that reads, "*These masks do not protect against the spread of infectious diseases.*" Did you get that? That is what we were mandated to do! Yet, they advertise that they don't protect you *right on the boxes! Are the people in authoritative positions smarter than your cells??*

Chapter 33
Antibodies and COVID-19?

You have been told antibodies are proteins made by the immune system to either fight off an illness or "remember" that we have encountered an "infectious" organism. The theory is before we encounter a virus or get sick from a virus, we have no antibodies to it. After getting sick, the PCR test should detect it. Here's the problem with that theory, it has no consistency, and it changes depending on the week. Also, have you noticed all the rules changed with this virus. You can be sick and have no antibodies, and you can be asymptomatic and positive. You can be negative and symptomatic. It's just a matter of what's needed for the outcome.

Remember when scientists used to tell you, you couldn't get a viral disease again once you had it due to your antibodies? Why did they stop? We guess that nonsense didn't fit their agenda of wanting to vaccinate you repeatedly.

Antibodies are proteins, and they support your body when it is removing toxins and repairing but *no scientific study shows they increase or decrease with a virus. Now THAT is big, no study shows antibodies increase or decrease with a virus.* They increase when you have been injected with something toxic! They increase when you have become toxic.

As for the production of antibodies and the immune system here are the results from one huge study, **"Immunity is a grand medical delusion**... In 1950, the British Medical Society conducted *exhaustive studies* on the relation of the incidence of diphtheria to the presence of antibodies. Their conclusion: **there is absolutely no relation between the two."** [90]

So, there you have it, an extensive study, and they found NO LINK and NO RELATION between antibodies and germs, bacteria, or viruses.

Antibodies, along with white blood cells and microorganisms, are involved in wound healing and cellular repair. However, their presence is not linked to any specific germ. There are absolutely no tests that indicate that antibodies are specific to anything.

Chapter 34
What's the deal with all the Vaccines? They're working, right?

We often come across the philosophical debates that ensue about vaccines. We call it philosophical, but it could also be termed *religious*. There is blind faith, so many people have in the power of vaccines to help their families stay healthy. So many have fallen for the mass deception; we hope we are convincing you *out* of it!

Mostly, often it is best to stay quiet and pretend you agree. No one wants to be labeled the dreaded "anti-vaxxer." The label is nothing short of being murderous and idiotic simultaneously. However, we can't even express the heartbreak that we have over the hundreds of people we know who have been affected by vaccine injury.

In the health profession, we hear our fair share of stories from taking the histories on patients. Still, the vaccine industry has a VERY good storyline they put on across all the media platforms based on the germ theory only. And once you know the secret of the germ theory fraud, the contagion fraud, and even the epidemic fraud, we hope you can consider the rest of these facts when you're making your future health decisions.

Chapter 35
Christine's Story

Let us tell you the heartbreaking story of Christine, who lost her daughter after being vaccinated. She writes, *"Death from vaccination is neither quick nor painless. I helplessly watched my daughter suffer an excruciatingly slow death as she screamed and arched her back in pain while the vaccine assaulted her immature immune system. The poisons used as preventatives seeped through her tiny body, overwhelming her vital organs one by one until they collapsed... My beautiful, innocent, infant daughter, death by lethal injection."* -Christine C.'s (her daughter died 24 hours after receiving a DPT shot.)

The real story began 150 years ago...

The idea behind vaccines was started in the 1800s. It's defined to produce immunity to a disease caused by a virus by using a "special preparation" to stimulate the production of appropriate antibodies. Therein lies the problem. *The vaccine "preparation" is always a mixture of horribly toxic substances to stimulate a reaction. Usually, the reaction is sickness. Initially, it was often death! Remember, we discovered in the private notes of Louis Pasteur that ALL 20 of his fully vaccinated experiment dogs DIED!!!*

Chapter 36
We have all heard that vaccinations save millions of lives.

Nothing could be further from the truth. We'll give you a brief history of the disaster that started as inoculations. In 1796 pus from cows was used in inoculations to "prevent disease". Originally pus from oozing cowpox sores was mixed with the blood of a healthy individual to create "freedom from disease." Although many died from this procedure and there were increased rates of smallpox in towns that used this procedure, it was used until 1840. Finally, "inoculations" were deemed too deadly!! They were discontinued due to the disastrous spread of smallpox *after inoculations*.

PF Colliers Encyclopedia, 1983- "As a rule, a certain percentage of fatalities and the contagiousness of the inoculated cases made the practice hazardous. Inoculation was prohibited in England in 1840." [91]

And then, as profiteering science would have it ...Along came the famous Edward Jenner.

Edward Jenner is regarded by the medical Industry as a hero (ironically) for his vaccine invention. He got his idea from a tale told by milkmaids that if you took the pus from cows inflicted with cowpox, they would have a less severe case of smallpox. He used this mixture with no known scientific experiments. He was paid very well.

Although Jenner is often called a physician, it is documented that he did not study for or pass the medical exam but purchased his medical degree. His qualification as a fellow of the Royal Society of England was not a result of any work related to medical matters but rather on the results of his study on the life of the *cuckoo bird!*

The only paper about vaccination that Jenner submitted to the Royal Society was rejected because it lacked proof. Other than his rejected paper, no further scientific work was submitted by Edward Jenner to the Royal Society for approval on vaccination.

Herbert Shelton explains: "Neither Jenner nor any of his successor's ever re-presented the claims for this vaccine, together with proofs to the Royal Society of England". But apparently, *belief in the cuckoo expert* was enough to roll out the vaccines.

In 1857, with no successful research, Edward Jenner got the smallpox "concoction" back out into the public with the new name of "Vaccinations". You must wonder, considering the year, whether he knew much of Louis Pasteur.

Chapter 37
Smallpox and the Medical Hippocratic Oath of "First do no harm?"

Smallpox is an acute disease that causes a fever and a rash that scars the skin. The medical establishment claims to have successfully eradicated this disease between the 1960s and 70s. However, history reveals that smallpox resided in cities due to overcrowding and sanitation issues. *It had nothing to do with the medical industry. As soon as hygiene and sanitation were implemented, smallpox disappeared.* Two cities, Cleveland, Ohio and Leicester, England both claim they became virtually free of smallpox by *abolishing vaccination* and increasing sanitation.

On the WHO website, it is quoted about the smallpox vaccine "no government gives or recommends smallpox vaccine routinely since it *can cause serious complications and even death.*"

When mandatory smallpox *vaccines were required* in 1867, there *were 57,016 smallpox deaths* between the years of 1871 and 1880. When vaccinations *were discontinued,* the total death rate from smallpox disease between 1911 and 1920 numbered only *110 total deaths.*

So much for smallpox vaccinations eradicating the disease of smallpox. The only true eradication comes from eradicating the vaccine!

Chapter 38
Goodbye Germ Theory!

In his incredible book, Good-bye Germ Theory, William Trebing has extensive research available to anyone. Here is the book briefly and some of his findings regarding vaccines.[92]

- "Smallpox would never have been the problem it was if the smallpox vaccine was not invented and promoted. In populations where there was no vaccine there was no smallpox."-1999; Glen Dettman, MD

- "Autism has increased by over 3000 times since the advent of mandatory vaccination programs, when it was considered very rare. The medical profession blames this on new diagnostic parameters, but this one cannot possibly have created such a drastic increase in so little time. The systematic blood poisoning of America's children through mercury and other products in vaccines is the only event which could possibly do this."

- "Following mandatory vaccine programs one of every 149 children in Brick Township, NJ is autistic."

- "Following mandatory vaccine programs between 1993 and 1998, autism increased 513% in the state of Maryland."

- "In India, between the years of 2010 and 2017 there have been over 490,000 children who have been paralyzed due to the oral polio vaccine! This fact was confirmed by two leading doctors in two reputable hospitals. Despite the government certified eradication of polio in India in 2011, the oral vaccine was given to millions of children by the Bill and Melinda Gates Foundation. -reported in newspaper, The Hindu, "Vaccine-induced paralysis calls for action, says study", by Bindu Shajan Perappandan

- "Also, studies from Finland and Turkey suggest that Guillain-Barré Syndrome (GBS) is causatively associated with Oral Polio vaccination campaigns."

- "Doctors are instructed by the American medical Association to downplay parents' concerns of vaccine reactions, and they deny any correlation of adverse reaction to vaccines they have just administered."

- "Federal government reports confirm the vaccinations kill more than three children per week in America."

- "Jonas Salk, creator of the famous Salk polio vaccine made a public statement in 1976 that 2/3 of the cases of polio which occurred between 1966 and 1976 were caused by his vaccine."

- "The DPT shot has been banned in most of Europe and Japan since 1975 due to its extreme toxicity, but American children still receive this vaccine."

- "Records prove the death rates from polio, pertussis, whooping cough and measles were decreasing on their own before the vaccines were introduced, and that present records were altered to demonstrate the decrease was due to vaccines."

- "Each year, they are approximately 950 deaths from the whooping cough vaccine as compared to 10 deaths from the actual disease."

- "Drug companies use the same pertussis shot to intentionally create encephalitis in experimental lab animals."

- "Over 95% of people who actually acquire diseases have been vaccinated against those very diseases! Drug companies refuse to study unvaccinated populations."

- "The "germ theory" does not follow any scientific guidelines to prove its validity. When assessed by the simple scientific method type in *elementary schools* it is proven invalid."

- "Pasteur's major credits do not belong to him but to another brilliant scientist called Pierre Bechamp, who totally disagreed with Pasteur's "germ theory" of disease creation. Most of Pasteur's early vaccine work ended in disaster."

- "The Center for Disease Control (CDC) charters an *epidemic intelligent service* which travels the country in search of symptoms they can use to formulate epidemics for profit! How disgusting is that?"

- "Most vaccination laws are completely unconstitutional and have no relevance to today's world. Local health departments promote most vaccine programs to acquire federal aid and grant money at the expense of America's children."

- "Everyone who wishes can enter a courtroom without the high cost of a lawyer, and WIN! You do not need to have to be vaccinated or to have your children vaccinated against your will. "

- "The FDA has reported the doctors under report vaccine reactions by 90%."

- "In any given population, the majority people who become ill are those who are vaccinated."

- "Unvaccinated populations can be proven scientifically and otherwise far healthier than vaccinated ones."

- "Encephalitis (brain damage due to the swelling in the brain tissue) is an almost given side effect of vaccine toxins according to most research studies on vaccine damages."

- "15 to 20% of American school children are considered to be learning disabled with brain damage dysfunction directly caused by vaccines."

- "Your government has paid over 4 billion in vaccination damage claims."

- "Your child is 94 times more likely to die from a whooping cough vaccine them from the actual whooping cough and nearly 4000 times more likely acquiring long-term damage from the vaccine then from developing the disease."

- "The CDC is aware that Thimerosal (Mercury preservative in vaccines) Is linked to autism by virtue of their own private research. However, they refused to provide the raw data from the studies, as requested by Congressman Dan Burton, to be used for an independent review by third-party research organization."

- "Giving a 10-pound infant a single vaccine in a day is the equivalent of giving 100-pound adult 40 vaccines in a day!"

- "Considering the above information, medical doctors insist on injecting 45 vaccines directly into your child's bloodstream by age 6 months; 64 by age 18 months; and 74 by age 6."

- "The CDC has an advisory committee on immunization practices called the ACIP. This committee advise lawmakers as to which vaccine should be mandated. ACIP is riddled with conflicts of interest, since committee members own patents for vaccines and stock in the pharmaceutical companies which make the vaccines."

- "Americans are amongst the most vaccinated people in the history of the planet and are also amongst the sickest in its history. 50% of all Americans suffer with at least one chronic disease, and 20% have 2 or more. These chronic diseases cause 70% of all American deaths." [92]

Chapter 39
What is the "Secret" revealed in plain sight?

Nature has supplied us with balance and harmony from the smallest particle of microzymas to the infinite cosmos. There is a hidden wealth of knowledge available to you whenever you choose to take responsibility for your health and look. It hides in plain sight to read, experience, and understand. It is also hidden within your common sense.

Germs are not meant to attack and destroy us, my friend. It is the opposite. It all goes back to spontaneous generation. You will produce germs you need when you need them. If you stay positive and let go of fears and resentment, your body and world will be filled with harmony!

Poisons and parasites attack our bodies, but GERMS don't. Poisons like King Cobra or Krate snake venom, Black Widow and Brown Recluse spider venom, Chemo drugs, Mustard Gas, and Chemical Warfare attack our cells and organs. Malaria and hookworms are parasites. As long as you haven't been poisoned or infected with a parasite, your body has every chance to heal quickly on its own. We should let go of old ideas that don't serve the truth.

You are made of stardust. It is time we all shine...

AFTERWORD - So where do we go from here?

This book reveals some hidden truths that will help you understand how wonderfully and divinely you are made by God. Nature has given you the gift of health and the ability to heal from disease. Disease does not come from bacteria, fungi, and viruses as the medical industry has forced on everyone. **Disease is a tissue manifestation or a tissue "response" that comes from specific programs that get triggered in a world of many situations perceived as threats to our survival. These threats are called "biological shocks or conflicts" in German New Medicine.** They are individual perceptions of our environment, and the brain and body tissue support us when we feel threatened. What we think of as germs and bacteria have evolved right along with our cells throughout our evolution *for a purpose*. The solution to our illnesses can be found in the cause. German New Medicine – the 5 Biological Laws Dr. Hamer discovered present us with answers and solutions to cancer and disease that truly work.

There are 120 disease programs clearly explained from the root cause to the healing stages by Dr. Ryke Hamer, MD.

There are many blogs by Isledora Laker on her site www.gnmonlineseminars.com. She is the CEO and main presenter at the GNM Institute of German New Medicine in Toronto, Canada.

These are amazing resources to help you understand the FUTURE OF MEDICINE is here now!

The Five Biological Laws of Nature – 5BN

Because German New Medicine (GNM) is Biological Medicine, what we think of as disease or cancer is called a Significant Biological Special Program (SBP).

First Biological Law of Nature Originally called "The Iron Rule of Cancer" *First criterion:* every Significant Biological Special Program (SBP) originates from a DHS (Dirk Hamer Syndrome), which is a serious, highly acute, dramatic, and isolating conflict shock that occurs simultaneously on three levels: psych–brain–organ.

Second criterion: DHS determines the location of the SBP both at brain level, the so-called Hammer Focus (HH), seen as concentric rings on a brain CT, and at the organ level, where it causes an organic alteration (what we commonly call a "disease"). Picture in your mind when a pebble drops in water. That is what the CT will show on the brain (and the organ!)

Third criterion: the course of the SBP runs synchronously on all three levels: psych–brain–organ, from the DHS (the conflict shock) to the resolution of the conflict (CL), including Epic-Crisis (EC) at the top (on a time line it is at the middle of the healing phase) of the Post Conflict Phase (PCL) until a normal level is restored (normatonia). More explanation of this can be found in the Second Law (see graph).

Second Biological Law of Nature

The law of two phases of all Significant Biological Special Programs (SBP) provided there is a resolution of the conflict (CL). Conflict Phase, considered the cold phase (CL), and a healing phase, considered the warm phase (PCL). During the second phase (PCL) there will be an

Epiletoid Crisis (EC) that can be a brief time or spike back into the conflict phase.

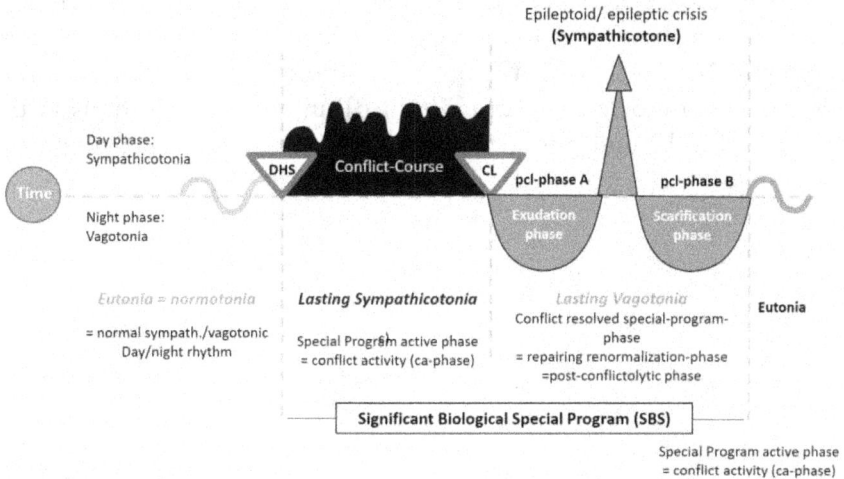

Third Biological Law of Nature

All SBP are directly related to the embryology of the human germ layers: Endoderm, Mesoderm, Ectoderm.

The ontogenetic system of Significant Biological Special Program (SBP) of cancer and cancer-equivalents, (cancer-SBP and cancer-equivalent-SBP). Cancer-equivalents are SBP without tumor and without ulcers, but with functional changes, for example, diabetes or M.S.

Fourth Biological Law of Nature

There is a correlation between the brain, the germ layers, and microbes. Microbes like mycobacteria, fungi, bacteria, and TB bacteria have a symbiotic relationship with our cells. Microbes breakdown and degrade overgrowths, or help build back cells during any cancer or disease process.

Fifth Biological Law of Nature: The "Quintessence"

Every so-called "disease" is part of a significant biological special program of nature, comprehensible in the context of our evolution.

The fifth biological natural law is the Quintessence of German New Medicine. It indicates that nothing in nature is meaningless or "malignant", as we have been taught. Each disease, DHS, that catches an individual "on the wrong foot" triggers a Significant Biological Special Program (SBP) which assist the organism in resolving the actual conflict situation. Even the "constellations" (2 SBP in opposite positions in the brain) can now be understood as meaningful, temporary meta-programs.

END NOTES

1 – *The Private Science of Louis Pasteur,* by Gerald Geisen

2 – https://en.m.wikipedia.org/wiki/Flat_Earth

3 – https://www.britannica.com/biography/Rudolf-Virchow

4 – The Truth About Contagion (Original title: The Contagion Myth) by Thomas S. Cowan, MD and Sally Fallon Morell

5 – The Truth About Contagion by Thomas S. Cowan, MD and Sally Fallon Morell p 5

6 – The Truth About Contagion by Thomas S. Cowan, MD and Sally Fallon Morell p 7

7 – *The Private Science of Louis Pasteur,* by Gerald Geisen, p 151

8 – Notes on Nursing, Florence Nightingale 1st ed. 1860 p.32

9 – What Really Makes You Ill? Why Everything You Thought You Knew About Disease is Wrong by Dawn Lester and David Parker.

10 – The Truth About Contagion by Thomas S. Cowan, MD and Sally Fallon Morell p 3, 4

11 – *The Private Science of Louis Pasteur,* by Gerald Geisen, p 181

12 – *The Private Science of Louis Pasteur,* by Gerald Geisen, p 157

13 – *The Private Science of Louis Pasteur,* by Gerald Geisen, p 241

14 – *The Private Science of Louis Pasteur,* by Gerald Geisen, p 251

15 – *The Private Science of Louis Pasteur,* by Gerald Geisen, p 198

16 – *The Private Science of Louis Pasteur,* by Gerald Geisen, p 242, 252

17 – *The Private Science of Louis Pasteur,* by Gerald Geisen, p 215

18 – *The Private Science of Louis Pasteur,* by Gerald Geisen, p 215

19 – The Truth About Contagion by Thomas S. Cowan, MD and Sally Fallon Morell p 4

20 – The Truth About Contagion by Thomas S. Cowan, MD and Sally Fallon Morell p 4

21 – Dr Stefan Lanka, Dr Andrew Kaufman, MD, Dr Thomas Cowan, MD, Dean Danes – Freedom Talk 5

22 – "The Real Anthony Fauci" Bill Gates, Big Pharma, and the Global War on Democracy and Public Health - by Robert F. Kennedy, Jr. pp 162, 173

23 – "The Real Anthony Fauci" Bill Gates, Big Pharma, and the Global War on Democracy and Public Health - by Robert F. Kennedy, Jr. pp 67

24 – VIRUS MANIA: Avian Flu (H5N1), Cervical Cancer (HPV), SARS, BSE, Hepatitis C, AIDS, Polio…How the Medical Industry Continually Invents Epidemics, Making Billion-Dollar Profits at Our Expense by Torsten Engelbrecht, Dr Claus Kohnlein, Dr Samantha Bailey, MD, Dr Stefano Scoglio, MD

25 – Electric Body, Electric Health by Eileen Day McKusick p 42

26 – Bechamp or Pasteur? By Ethel Hume p 243

27 – Bechamp or Pasteur? A Lost Chapter in the History of Biology, By Ethel Hume 1919 and Pasteur: Plagiarist, Imposter; The Germ theory Exploded by R.B. Pearson 1942 Note from the publisher of both books admin@adistantmirror.com.au 2017.

28 – Pasteur: Plagiarist and Imposter; The Germ Theory Exploded, 1942, p 30

29 – Pasteur: Plagiarist and Imposter; The Germ Theory Exploded, 1942, p 28

30 – "All go to the same place; all came from the *dust*, and all return to the *dust*." - Ecclesiastes 3:20

31 – https://www.britannica.com/biography/Rudolf-Virchow

32 – Bechamp or Pasteur? By Ethel Hume p 245

33 – Dr. William Trebing, Goodbye Germ Theory p 151

34 – 2002 textbook Molecular Biology of the Cell

35 – Notes on Nursing, Florence Nightingale 1st ed. 1860 and

Pasteur: Plagiarist, Imposter The Germ Theory Exploded by R. B. Pearson p 13

36 – Dr. William Trebing, Goodbye Germ Theory p 155

37 – Dr. William Trebing, Goodbye Germ Theory p 155

38 – Dr. William Trebing, Goodbye Germ Theory p 154

39 – www.Learninggnm.com

40 – www.learninggnm.com, Caroline Markolin, PhD

41 – 1921 by the *Hygienic Laboratory #123* https://www.scribd.com/document/578758384/20210424-Spanische-Grippe-Studie

42 – andrewkaufmanmd.co

43 – Co-Senior Investigato1r, Ken Caldwell, PhD.

44 – Dec 9, 2019, Report: What Are Exosomes and Why are They Important

45 – Dr. Wu Zunyou, MD, PhD, is the Chief Epidemiologist of Chinese Center for Disease Control and Prevention, and an Adjunct Professor of Epidemiology at University of California at Los Angeles.

46 – "The Real Anthony Fauci" Bill Gates, Big Pharma, and the Global War on Democracy and Public Health by Robert F. Kennedy, Jr. pp 126

47 – Event 201: October 2019 "The Real Anthony Fauci" Bill Gates, Big Pharma, and the Global War on Democracy and Public Health by Robert F. Kennedy, Jr. pp 402-425, 434.

48 – CPE - Control Experiment - 21 April 2021 - English version (odysee.com)

https://odysee.com/@DeansDanes:1/cpe-english:f

49 – VIRUS MANIA: Avian Flu (H5N1), Cervical Cancer (HPV), SARS, BSE, Hepatitis C, AIDS, Polio…How the Medical Industry Continually Invents Epidemics, Making Billion-Dollar Profits at Our Expense by Torsten Engelbrecht, Dr Claus Kohnlein, Dr Samantha Bailey, MD, Dr Stefano Scoglio, MD

50 – What Really Makes You Ill? Why Everything You Thought You Knew About Disease is Wrong by Dawn Lester and David Parker p 89

51 – Confessions of a Medical Heretic by Dr. Robert Mendelsohn, MD

52 – Symbiotic Planet by Dr Margulis

53 – Goodbye Germ Theory by Dr William Trebing p 155

54 – What Really Makes You Ill? Why Everything You Thought You Knew About Disease is Wrong by Dawn Lester and David Parker p 53

55 – What Really Makes You Ill? Why Everything You Thought You Knew About Disease is Wrong by Dawn Lester and David Parker p 54

56 – 1948 John Paul of Yale University, International Poliomyelitis Congress

57 – 1941 Scientific Journal ARCHIVES of Pediatrics

58 – May 1955 Carl Eklund

59 – Fear of the Invisible: A Hidden Epidemic by Janine Roberts p 66

60 – Fear of the Invisible: A Hidden Epidemic by Janine Roberts p 66

61 – Vaccination, Greg Beattie p 53

62 – Virus Mania, Good-bye Germ Theory, What Really makes you sick

63 – What Really Makes You Ill? Why Everything You Thought You Knew About Disease is Wrong by Dawn Lester and David Parker p 54

64 – Invisible Rainbow by Arthur Firstenberg p 107

65 – Vaccine Whistleblower: Exposing Autism Research Fraud at the CDC by Kevin Barry

66 – VIRUS MANIA: Avian Flu (H5N1), Cervical Cancer (HPV), SARS, BSE, Hepatitis C, AIDS, Polio…How the Medical Industry Continually Invents Epidemics, Making Billion-Dollar Profits at Our Expense by Torsten Engelbrecht, Dr Claus Kohnlein, Dr Samantha Bailey, MD, Dr Stefano Scoglio, MD pp 90-152

67 –Dr. Heinz Ludwig Sanger, Emeritus Professor of Molecular Biology and Virology, Max-Planck-Institute for Biochemistry, Munich

68 – Vaccination - Genocide in the third Millennium? By Stefan Lanka and Karl Krafeld read more at: https://www.preciousorganics.com.au/pages/dr-stefan-lanka-exposes-the-viral-fraud

69 – http://www.virusmyth.com/aids/controversy.htm

70 – *Reinharth Kurth*, director of the Robert Koch Institute in Der Speigel, September 9th, 2004

71 – Goodbye Germ Theory by Dr William Trebing p 159

72 – Goodbye Germ Theory by Dr William Trebing p 159

73 – VIRUS MANIA: Avian Flu (H5N1), Cervical Cancer (HPV), SARS, BSE, Hepatitis C, AIDS, Polio…How the Medical Industry Continually Invents Epidemics, Making Billion-Dollar Profits at Our Expense by Torsten Engelbrecht, Dr Claus Kohnlein, Dr Samantha Bailey, MD, Dr Stefano Scoglio, MD p 161-164

74 – "The Real Anthony Fauci" Bill Gates, Big Pharma, and the Global War on Democracy and Public Health - by Robert F. Kennedy, Jr.

75 – www.Learninggnm.com

76 – VIRUS MANIA: Avian Flu (H5N1), Cervical Cancer (HPV), SARS, BSE, Hepatitis C, AIDS, Polio…How the Medical Industry

Continually Invents Epidemics, Making Billion-Dollar Profits at Our Expense by Torsten Engelbrecht, Dr Claus Kohnlein, Dr Samantha Bailey, MD, Dr Stefano Scoglio, MD p 116

77 – Haverkos, Harry, Disease Manifestation among Homosexual Men with Acquired Immunodeficiency Syndrome: A Possible Role of Nitrites in Kaposi's Sarcoma, *Sexually Transmitted Diseases*, October- December 1985, pp. 203-208

78 – Krieger, Terry; Caceres, Cesar; *The Unnoticed Link in AIDS cases*, Wall Street Journal, 24 October 1985

79 – VIRUS MANIA: Avian Flu (H5N1), Cervical Cancer (HPV), SARS, BSE, Hepatitis C, AIDS, Polio…How the Medical Industry Continually Invents Epidemics, Making Billion-Dollar Profits at Our Expense by Torsten Engelbrecht, Dr Claus Kohnlein, Dr Samantha Bailey, MD, Dr Stefano Scoglio, MD p 103

80 – VIRUS MANIA: Avian Flu (H5N1), Cervical Cancer (HPV), SARS, BSE, Hepatitis C, AIDS, Polio…How the Medical Industry Continually Invents Epidemics, Making Billion-Dollar Profits at Our Expense by Torsten Engelbrecht, Dr Claus Kohnlein, Dr Samantha Bailey, MD, Dr Stefano Scoglio, MD p 167

81 – VIRUS MANIA: Avian Flu (H5N1), Cervical Cancer (HPV), SARS, BSE, Hepatitis C, AIDS, Polio…How the Medical Industry Continually Invents Epidemics, Making Billion-Dollar Profits at Our Expense by Torsten Engelbrecht, Dr Claus Kohnlein, Dr Samantha Bailey, MD, Dr Stefano Scoglio, MD p 166-167

82 – Dr. William Trebing, Goodbye Germ Theory P 161

83 – VIRUS MANIA: Avian Flu (H5N1), Cervical Cancer (HPV), SARS, BSE, Hepatitis C, AIDS, Polio…How the Medical Industry Continually Invents Epidemics, Making Billion-Dollar Profits at Our Expense by Torsten Engelbrecht, Dr Claus Kohnlein, Dr Samantha Bailey, MD, Dr Stefano Scoglio, MD p 159

84 – Dr. Stefan Lanka: "All claims about viruses as pathogens are false" report.

85 – www.Rumble.com Scoundrel Weapon Information Distribution Channel June 24, 2021

86 – The Truth About Contagion by Thomas S. Cowan, MD and Sally Fallon Morell p 51

87 – The Truth About Contagion by Thomas S. Cowan, MD and Sally Fallon Morell p 51

88 – Kary Mullis Interview
https://www.youtube.com/watch?v=RE0e7gj6x20

89 – "The Real Anthony Fauci" Bill Gates, Big Pharma, and the Global War on Democracy and Public Health by Robert F. Kennedy, Jr. p 446

90 – There's more to Vaccination than the Shot By Sharon Kimmelman

91 – PF Colliers Encyclopedia, 1983

92 – Good-bye Germ Theory, William Trebing

93 – Five Biological Laws of Nature – 5BN – Scientific Chart of German New Medicine by Dr. med. Mag. Theol. Ryke Geerd Hamer; 5 Biological Laws and Dr. Hamer's New Medicine by Andrea Taddei

BIOGRAPHIES

Dr. Robert DeSantis grew up in Bozeman, Montana. He had a large wellness practice for over 30 years in the northwest region of Washington state. There he taught thousands of people healing and wellness principles. Dr. DeSantis has been committed to helping patients establish their own self-healing techniques. He is committed to helping people understand the body's divine ability for self-healing. He has been researching mind, body and soul principles for over 45 years. Dr. DeSantis lives in the Midwest of the United States with his two daughters and dog.

David Lloyd has been an educator since 1988. He has a degree in Education and Music. He is also a creative writer, poet, musician, Yoga Teacher, Reiki Master, and CECP (Certified Emotion Code Practitioner) through Discover Healing and Dr. Bradley Nelson, D.C.

He has completed the Intermediate GNM Course for Medical Professionals through The GNM Institute in Toronto, Canada, and is completing the Advanced Clinician's Program.